PHENOMENOLOGY OF THE NEWBORN

Many children spend their first days, weeks, and sometimes months in a neonatal intensive care unit as a consequence of prematurity, congenital anomalies, or birth complications. Their medical needs are thoughtfully appraised and attended to, yet some questions are rarely asked: What experiences do these newborns have? What experiences are we giving them? How can we and do we understand what their lives are like? What are the interventions and actions of medical care actually like for them?

Michael van Manen explores the experiential life of newborn infants with particular consideration for those newborns who require medical care. Drawing on contemporary research findings from physiology, psychology, biology, and other disciplines, he offers phenomenological insights and raises thought-provoking questions as to how we ought to understand and care for such young children.

In our contemporary world, it is often the experiences of inception, of first contact, with those who seem most distant, foreign, or even alien that we need to try to apprehend and understand. The inceptual lives of newborn infants challenges us to explore those experiences phenomenologically—to investigate the originary meanings of early life experiences. *Phenomenology of the Newborn* is an essential text for researchers seeking to employ phenomenology for the study of neonatal life and related concerns that may seem inaccessible to other more traditional qualitative and quantitative methods.

Michael van Manen, MD, PhD, is an Assistant Professor in the Department of Paediatrics, Faculty of Medicine and Dentistry, University of Alberta, Canada. He has a clinical practice as a physician in neonatal-perinatal medicine with the Stollery Children's Hospital.

PHENOMENOLOGY OF PRACTICE

Series editor: Max van Manen, *University of Alberta*, Canada

The series Phenomenology of Practice sponsors books that are steeped in phenomenological scholarship and relevant to professional practitioners in fields such as education, nursing, medicine, pedagogy, clinical and counseling psychology. Texts in this series distinguish themselves for offering inceptual and meaningful insights into lived experiences of professional practices, or into the quotidian concerns of everyday living. Texts may reflectively explicate and focus on aspects of method and dimensions of the philosophic and human science underpinnings of phenomenological research.

For further manuscript details available from the Series Editor please contact Max van Manen at vanmanen@ualberta.ca / +250-294 4345

Other volumes in this series include:

Visual Phenomenology
Encountering the Sublime Through Images
Erika Goble

Pedagogical Tact
Knowing What to Do When You Don't Know What to Do
Max van Manen

For a full list of titles in this series, please visit https://www.routledge.com/Phenomenology-of-Practice/book-series/PPVM

PHENOMENOLOGY OF THE NEWBORN

Life from Womb to World

Michael van Manen

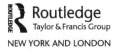

Routledge
Taylor & Francis Group

NEW YORK AND LONDON

First published 2019
by Routledge
52 Vanderbilt Avenue, New York, NY 10017

and by Routledge
2 Park Square, Milton Park, Abingdon, Oxon OX14 4RN

Routledge is an imprint of the Taylor & Francis Group, an informa business

© 2019 Taylor & Francis

Chapter 2 is based on article published: van Manen, M. (2017). Towards the
womb of neonatal intensive care. *Journal of Medical Humanities*. doi:10.1007/
s10912–017–9494–9
Chapter 3 is based on article published: van Manen, M. (2017). The first cry of
the child. *Qualitative Health Research*, 27(7), 1069–1076. doi:10.1177/
1049732316673342

Library of Congress Cataloging-in-Publication Data
Names: Van Manen, Michael, author.
Title: Phenomenology of the newborn : life from womb to world /
Michael van Manen.
Other titles: Phenomenology of practice (Routledge (Firm))
Description: New York, NY : Routledge, 2019. |
Series: Phenomenology of practice | Includes bibliographical references.
Identifiers: LCCN 2018031654| ISBN 9781138486362 (hbk) |
ISBN 9781138486379 (pbk) | ISBN 9781351045674 (ebk)
Subjects: | MESH: Infant, Newborn | Consciousness | Infant, Newborn,
Diseases--psychology | Philosophy, Medical
Classification: LCC RJ254 | NLM WS 420 | DDC 618.92/01--dc23
LC record available at https://lccn.loc.gov/2018031654

ISBN: 978-1-138-48636-2 (hbk)
ISBN: 978-1-138-48637-9 (pbk)
ISBN: 978-1-351-04567-4 (ebk)

Typeset in Bembo
by Taylor & Francis Books

For my mother and father

CONTENTS

ACKNOWLEDGEMENTS

I would like to thank the parents and families for their willingness to participate in these studies of care of their newborns, especially when conditions and circumstances were sometimes very difficult and demanding. It is a great privilege, as a practicing neonatal physician, along with the parents, to look after each unique child with his or her unique possibilities. I also thank the practicing trainees, bedside nurses, respiratory therapists, dieticians, pharmacists, social workers, nurse practitioners, and colleague physicians in Neonatal-Perinatal Medicine at the Stollery Children's Hospital for their support. In sharing their experiences, thoughts, and reflections, they contributed greatly to this work. I thank my amazing wife, Miep, for her support and love, as well as my children, Luka and Jude, for their inspiration. I am appreciative of my colleagues at the John Dossetor Health Ethics Centre. I thank Kristy Wolfe for her skill and sensitivity in photographing the babies pictured in this book, and the parents for granting permission to include the images. I am grateful for the funding received from the Canadian Institutes for Health Research and the Women & Children's Health Research Institute that made this work possible. This book aims to understand how to best serve newborns in their challenges, as they each transition in their own way from the womb into the world. So, finally, my deepest "thank you" is to each newborn: You may not yet realize the weight and significance of this "thank you" but this is about you and for you.

PREFACE

Within the womb stirs life's beginnings: a yet-to-be-born child shifts in position before slowly straightening a foot. The expectant mother holds her hand against her belly. She feels the movement, a localized pressure or a vague fullness. While she may give the stirring little thought in that particular moment, perhaps she touches her belly in a searching way: feeling to feel a sensation that she can identify as a push, a stretch, or a kick. Or perhaps she recognizes the movement as a touch of her child, touching her in response to her hand. As the weeks of pregnancy progress we may wonder: how sensate is the unborn him- or herself in such moments? What feeling if any might the fetus feel? If the mother were not to pause and not to touch her abdomen, would there be different consequences for her child?

Months pass, marked by moments of activity and relative calmness, until the day of birth arrives. It is on this birth day that a baby is born into the world. Somehow, during this inceptual time of the pregnancy, the fetal body-brain gave birth to a primal consciousness. But what is the nature of this initial wombed awareness or unawareness? And how does it enter by birth to the world? Our first thought may be that for the newborn the exterior world is full of foreign sounds, smells, lights, and other strange sensations. However, we may witness that when the baby is brought to its mother to settle against her chest there is no observable sense of foreignness or strangeness. The arms and legs still as mother and child are skin-to-skin. And then the pace of life resumes as the baby slowly shifts in position and, as before, straightens a foot.

Yet, there are other children whose lives outside the womb start ever so differently. Many children spend their first days, weeks, and sometimes months in a neonatal intensive care unit (NICU). In developed countries, approximately one in ten babies are born premature (World Health Organization, 2018), and despite advances in medical care, children continue to be born with complications such as birth asphyxia or require protracted hospital stays for treatment of congenital anomalies (Dukhovny et al., 2016). Much care is given to these children. Their medical needs are thoughtfully appraised and attended. Yet, some questions are rarely asked: What experiences do these newborns have? What experiences are we giving them? How can we and do we understand what their lives are like? What are the interventions and actions of intensive care actually like for newborns?

Surely, we may find ourselves emotionally stirred when first faced with the image, description, or story of a hospitalized newborn who lies vulnerable and exposed in a neonatal isolette, hooked up to various clinical, technological equipment. But the critical challenge for healthcare professionals is that if we are asked what these children actually experience, we find ourselves strangely speechless. We do not really know. Our understanding of the experiential life of a newborn is always already framed from a perspective of distance and reflectiveness. Although we have all been newborns, we simply cannot recall or even imagine our first days of life; these events seem too remotely buried in our past. And even if we could reconstitute our early existence, is our vocabulary, let alone our understanding, really true and suited to recapture the life of a newborn? Are adult interpretive sensibilities of pain, distress, comfort, and pleasure appropriately attuned in describing a newborn's experience? Might newborns experience the world somehow in a more elusively original, primal, or less differentiated manner than adults do and can comprehend? These are crucial questions for frontline practitioners who work in neonatal-perinatal medicine and related fields. Physicians and nurses may need to answer what are the expected consequences for the child of being born premature, enduring medical tests, and/or undergoing surgical procedures. What understanding do we have of the lives of newborns? How are understandings conditioned by medical practice, technologies, or other affordances? How do we support a newborn to be realized as a child?

It may sound strange, but physicians, nurses, and other healthcare professionals need to orient themselves and sensitize others to the NICU newborn's childness. How we converse with parents about an infant born with a congenital anomaly may ameliorate sensitivity to the newborn as a child if the conversation is purely focused on the medical details of a diagnosis and treatment. Similarly, a premature infant may be understood as premature in his or her childness, not quite a child yet. There is the risk of fostering a feeling of distance from these children. For the brain-injured child, we need to consider how we present parents with a possible view of the future life that may be complicated by disabilities or medical consequences. In this way, healthcare professionals may exert significant effects on the unfolding relationship between parents and their newborns. This is the ethics of neonatology: how healthcare professionals help bring the newborn as a child from the womb into the world.

Contemporary empirical studies from the fields of physiology, psychology, and other scientific disciplines provide suggestive and tentative evidence that some experiential consciousness of the world may dawn and develop within the womb even prior to birth. How this experiential existence is comparable to the conscious awareness or unawareness of the older child or adult, however, remains an enigma. Even so, the fetal behavior literature reveals that the womb is a place of sensate existence, and that it is formative of impending activities and perceptions. Researchers recognize that newborns already possess complex albeit developing cognitive capacities. Medical and other caring professions increasingly realize the importance of considering the quality of sensory experiences of infants who require NICU care. And yet, we are only beginning to discern meaningful understandings as to how fetal and neonatal impressions may coalesce and develop over time.

The aim of this book is to explore the experiential life of the newborn, with particular consideration for newborns requiring medical care in a NICU. The life of the newborn is approached from a phenomenological orientation. Phenomenology is the study of human experience itself, and the meanings that are given in experience. The intent is not to generate theory so much as to explore possible understandings and insights into what constitutes experiential life. Such understandings require special methodological sources. For the world of the newborn, we need to draw on findings from empirical research.

Examining empirical research data from a phenomenological perspective is a form of *constative* reflecting: uncovering plausible truths, against a constant background of unknowing and wonder. How is current medical care attentive to the sensory experiences of infants? What moments of meaningfulness do premature infants experience? In what way should we attend to these infants who are born prematurely from the womb? A wondering reflection may give us constatations: insights that possess not empirical certainty, but phenomenological plausibility, a probing *veritas*, or *alethea*.

The philosopher Marion (2002) points out that the birth of a baby has obvious meaning, making possible and anticipating all experiences to come, and yet the subjectivity of this profound event cannot be simply remembered or recalled. Still, when watching, touching, holding, and quite simply being with newborns we may find ourselves stirred as we have a primal awareness of the miraculous meaningfulness of a life coming to *life*. We sense the affectivity of life that surges through existence—an existence we share with this newborn newcomer. This encounter with the beginning of a life unfolding into subjectivity and consciousness occurs in the field of neonatology, the subspecialty of pediatrics that consists in the medical care and safeguarding of the new infant life as it has left the womb. Neonatology specializes in the care for premature and ill newborns— usually practiced in NICUs.

This book features two methodological chapters and six phenomenological studies. Chapters may be read in isolation though they have been arranged with the aim of introducing the reader to the life of the newborn transitioning from womb to world. Healthcare professional readers may choose to start with Chapter 2 rather than dwell on methodological issues introduced in Chapter 1. Still, I have endeavored to write each chapter in an accessible manner, regardless of a reader's background in phenomenological inquiry.

The focus of Chapter 1 is on phenomenology as a method of human science inquiry. While there exist exemplary texts on phenomenological research (see Giorgi, 1970, 2009; van Manen, 1990, 2014), methods to explore the lived experiences of infants, children, and adults, who are unable to describe and reflect on their own experiences, have received limited attention. Indeed, the life of a newborn is a paradigm case for phenomenological human science inquiry. Infancy, from the Latin *infantem*, means "not able to speak" (*OED*). Phenomenological inquiry explores human experience of being-in-the-world, recognizing that our lived through experiences may be subtle and elusive, ambiguous and complex. In this chapter, key phenomenological notions such as lived experience, subjectivity, and intersubjectivity are introduced with the intent of examining the meaning interpretations of observational accounts of infant behavior. As well, some methodological issues are considered for using experimental observations or other such findings of empirical research in service of phenomenological inquiry. Subsequent chapters provide examples, studies, of the application of a phenomenological method to explore possible subjective experiences of newborn life.

Chapter 2 opens with the question of the inception of experiential human life, focusing on the conditions and paths of 'becoming' for the fetus within the womb. This chapter is an important starting point for all subsequent chapters, recognizing that in the study of the life of the newborn we need to ask when might experiential sensibility and consciousness actually begin, and what might compose its sensuality? The implications of caring for children born prematurely (from the womb) who require neonatal intensive care are also explored to show the striking differences in environmental sensuality between the womb and the NICU. Such explorations are important to determine the ethical implications of established and emerging NICU care practices. Methodologically, this chapter is an example of engaging primarily with embryological, developmental, and behavioral research to explore the lived meaning of a phenomenon.

Chapter 3 explores the phenomenon of the first cry of the newly born child. The first cry is an important occurrence as it signals that a uniquely separate life has begun, the transition from womb to world life. Although the phenomenon of the first cry may be functionally explained from evolutionary, psychological, or physiological perspectives, a phenomenological method questions the meaning of the first cry as an expression of the assumed unsettling nature of the birthing event. How is the first cry experienced by the birthing mother and attending adults? What is the possible meaning of the first cry for the newborn infant? Pedagogical questions are raised related to how we may understand and respond to well and sick newborns in their crying. Methodologically, this chapter is an example of engaging primarily with physiological and observational research to explore the lived meaning of a phenomenon.

Chapter 4 explores the experiential life of the child born prematurely. The construct 'disorganized behavior' (as described in the Synactive Theory of Development literature, the theoretical basis of the internationally recognized Newborn Developmental Care and Assessment Program) is used as a starting point for reflection. Phenomenology questions whether there is in fact order to this disorder as lacking contact, unsettling stimulation, and exposed bodiliness. This chapter examines the ethics of using a behavioral language when providing developmental care to infants in the NICU. It asks what are we inclined to miss in our understanding and practice when an infant's experience is framed by and conceptualized in a behavioral paradigm. Methodologically, this chapter is an example of engaging primarily with behavioral observations to explore the lived meaning of a phenomenon.

Chapter 5 explores our personal, adult, intersubjective relations with newborns, taking the newborn gaze as an event that may awaken our awareness to the consciousness of the conscious being of an infant. This chapter also considers how the newborn's body as torso, hands, feet, and mouth are perceptually active in a contacting way. This relational inquiry explores the possibility of the health professional being aware of the infant 'seeing' in all manner of moments, yet also cautioning the reader that such awareness must reflect a questioning attitude. Methodologically, this chapter uses images and anecdotes to explore the lived meaning of a phenomenon, a lived experience or event.

Chapter 6 explores the possibility for infants to experience adult interpretive sensibilities of pain, anxiety, and other experiences of distress, and the meanings that may inhere in languages pertaining to newborns. This chapter questions established medical practices of assessing infants, and in particular the widespread use of pain and agitation scales. This concern is particularly relevant to physicians, nurses, and other healthcare professionals as they engage in medical dialogue with respect to infant experience, and how decisions are made with respect to the use of analgesic-sedative medications and other care measures. Methodologically, this chapter is an example of engaging primarily with narrative, psychological, and observational research to explore the lived meaning of a phenomenon.

Chapter 7 explores the newborn baby suckle in its ordinary and extraordinary existential significance. To feed is a basic capacity of every healthy newborn child, and from this everyday act, newborn consciousness may be investigated. Such inquiry is again brought back to questions about the nature of the experiential being of the newborn who requires care in a NICU where feeding may need to be adjusted and compromised in the context of prematurity or medical illness. Methodologically, this chapter is an example of engaging primarily with physiological and observational research to explore the lived meaning of a phenomenon.

Chapter 8 aims at gathering the themes of the previous chapters by articulating the ethical significance and value of exploring the experiential life of the newborn, with particular attention to infants requiring medical care. This chapter discusses the necessity for a phenomenology of practice to respond to the challenge of researching the lived experiences of infants or those who are 'not able to speak' in ways we can directly comprehend.

Research into the experiential lives of infants is very much in its infancy: not yet able to speak fully of its enigmatic subject of infant subjectivity. This work may be judged as successful if it stimulates the reader's wondering, thoughtfulness, and sensitivity to the world of hospitalized newborns. My hope is that this book not only serves parents and healthcare professionals concerned with the wellbeing of newborns, but also that it provides examples for those seeking to employ phenomenology to research experiences that may seem inaccessible to other qualitative and quantitative methods. In our contemporary world, it is often the experiences of inception, of first contact, with those who seem most distant, foreign, or even alien that we need to apprehend and understand.

References

Dukhovny, D., Pursley, D. M., Kirpalani, H. M., Horbar, J. H., & Zupancic, J. A. (2016). "Evidence, quality, and waste: solving the value equation in neonatology." *Pediatrics*, 137(3), e20150312.

Giorgi, A. (1970). *Psychology as a Human Science: A Phenomenologically Based Approach*. New York, NY: Harper & Row.

Giorgi, A. (2009). *The Descriptive Phenomenological Method in Psychology: A Modified Husserlian Approach*. Pittsburgh, PA: Duquesne University Press.

Marion, J-L. (2002). *In Excess: Studies of Saturated Phenomenon*. (R. Horner, V. Berrand, transl.) New York, NY: Fordham University Press. (Original work published 2001).

Van Manen, M. (1990). *Researching Lived Experience: Human Science for an Action Sensitive Pedagogy*. Albany, NY: SUNY Press; London, ON: Althouse Press.

Van Manen, M. (2014). *Phenomenology of Practice: Meaning-Giving Methods in Phenomenological Research and Writing*. Walnut Creek, CA: Left Coast Press.

World Health Organization. (2018). Preterm birth. Fact sheet. Updated February 2018. Retrieved from www.who.int/en/news-room/fact-sheets/detail/preterm-birth.

1

INCEPTUAL QUESTIONS

The study of newborn existence raises questions as to whether fundamental philosophical notions actually apply to the experiential world of the newborn. Are terms such as 'lived experience,' 'consciousness,' 'subjectivity,' and 'intersubjectivity' appropriate for describing a newborn's existence? How can phenomenological inquiry proceed without being confident of the language we use? What considerations need to be given to the method of phenomenology for empathically approaching or accessing the world of the newborn?

A newborn is likely to experience the world in a vastly different mode than an older child or adult owing to differences in body-brain maturity and the pure temporality of natality. And yet, as adults we do have understandings, or at the very least, we carry out our day-to-day activities interacting with newborns with an assumed sense as to why they fuss, cry, sooth, settle, or otherwise act within and respond to the world. A phenomenology of the newborn explores such understandings not by an ethereal exploration above and beyond the way a newborn's body and brain function, but instead by attentiveness to the knowledge that empirical sciences have generated— importantly, phenomenology is also alert to the philosophical presumptions underlying such knowledge.

Contemporary empirical infancy research shows that newborns come to possess complex, cognitive competencies that exceed their overt everyday actions (Rochat, 2001). Such research has the potential to inform our understanding of the newborn's world as inhabited. Still, empirical researchers may all too readily lose sight of the lived meaning of newborn experiences by instead focusing on newborn behavioral development from an objectifying perspective—a perspective that sees newborns primarily as immature in their development. In other words, rather than wonder what a newborn's subjective and inner life may be like, it focuses instead on the developmental accomplishments achieved by an infant from an external perspective.

What Constitutes the Lived Existence of a Newborn?

A premature baby has been placed in an isolette (a neonatal incubator). A sheet cast over the housing mutes ambient light just as the plastic structure itself attenuates sound. Only traces of the outside world seem to be allowed in. Within the isolette, rolled towels support the baby's body in a position of flexion. The arms, torso, and legs shift in subtle shutters before settling in stillness. Eyes gaze, yet seem to lack a point of fixation.

What is life within the isolette like for this child? While it might be assumed that this premature infant is unaware of its external and internal ambience, this assumption is unwarranted. Do the gazing eyes not see? Does the fidgeting body not feel? What sensibility may actually be present in this baby? And, what words are appropriate to describe his or her existence?

For phenomenology, the term 'lived experience' signifies the living through-ness of each moment of our existence. The "phenomenological thesis" says that experience is first and foremost pre-reflective, pre-predicative, and pre-linguistic (Romano, 2015, p. xi). For the most part, we do not think about our experiences as we live through them. This does not mean that our experiences are not meaningful, but rather that we do not reflectively dwell on these meanings while we are experiencing them. Our ordinary everyday lived experiences are largely taken-for-granted as we are absorbed in the ongoing happenings of our lives.

At times an event may prompt a pause, notice, or reflection. And in such contemplative moments, we may become aware of how meaningful a moment in our lives was. The point is that such meaning, which is at the heart of experience, is always already there, founded in the way we directly experience being-in-the-world as lived experience. For example, when a loved one shares in conversation the occurrences of their day, we nod both to confirm we understand the matter-of-fact happenings surrounding an event and also the meaningfulness of an event. We understand terms such as annoying, frustrating, invigorating, satisfying, and so forth because we appreciate the meanings that inhere in the experiences even before such terms are used to describe emotive reactions or feelings. While we cannot hazard if the fetus or newborn has contemplative capacities, we should wonder what meanings constitute their lived existence. We wonder how a newborn directly experiences the world.

The assumption and belief that the newborn experiences the world without meaning has already been largely disproved. We can simply no longer accept that the newborn "feels it all as one great blooming, buzzing confusion" as described over a century ago by William James (1890, p. 488). Research has shown that the newborn may already orient to differing smells (Marlier & Schaal, 2005; Marlier et al., 2007), sounds (DeCasper & Fifer, 1980), and touches (Butterworth & Hopkins, 1988; Rochat & Hespos, 1997; Rochat et al., 1988) in their distinctiveness. And yet the discovery that a newborn discriminates between smells, sounds, and touches does not answer what meanings reside in such discriminating sensuality.

The challenge to access the experiential world of the newborn, or even an older child or adult, is that we need to somehow turn towards experience as meaning arises (as it is lived through). Yet, as soon as we try to introspect an experiential moment, it becomes objectified by our reflective glance. If we try to attend to an experience as we live through it, the lived through experience itself cannot help but be changed to an experience of reflecting. We can only retrospect the meaning of experiences. So, if we aim to capture an experience after we have lived through it, we are always already too late. Similarly, by analogy, we tend to objectify a newborn's experiential world by using words such as agitation or distress. A phenomenological, reflective glance aims to understand a living moment of existence.

> [R]eflection is not at all the noting of a fact. It is, rather, an attempt to understand. It is not the passive attitude of a subject who watches himself live but rather the active effort of a subject who grasps the meaning of his experience.
>
> *(Merleau-Ponty, 1964a, p. 64)*

Reflecting phenomenologically on experience is not an act of abstraction, conceptualization, or theory generation; nor an endeavor of self-analysis, meditation, or soul-searching. Rather, it is an effortful questioning of experience, engaging with our own existent sensibilities, gaining an experiential grasp of being-in-the-world.

In so far as we can appreciate or recognize an experience as resonant with our sensibilities, phenomenological inquiry aims to bring these sensibilities to concrete, experiential understanding. But this understanding encompasses more than expressible propositions, statements, or facts. There are primal meanings to experiences that may be ambiguous, indistinct, or simply resistant to articulate in their primality (Ricoeur, 1966, p. 208). As adults we can reflect on an experience of a moment of pain or anguish, delight or joy, or any other stretch of experience. Yet, we may have a hard time articulating or finding words that adequately describe such lived experience even if the experience is our own. There is always something about an experience that may evade reflection: there always remains a difference between the lived and the articulated (Merleau-Ponty, 1962, p. 393). The lived meanings of lived experience are subtle and elusive, ambiguous and complex. This pre-reflectivity of lived experience is a challenge to our efforts to bring experience to language.

> Phenomenology is not as naïve as some people pretend. It does not presuppose that what appears is completely outside of language, but it does presuppose that what happens and appears to us is more than what can be

said about it and what can be argued for or against it. The crucial point is not to assume that there is something given outside of language, but to concede that language precedes itself.

(Waldenfels, 2007, p. 88)

The language of phenomenological reflection attends to the manner in which an experience is given to consciousness, to gently lift that which otherwise may be readily passed over by awareness to (re)call the experience to presence. We must ultimately name or bring to language meanings as they are experienced, recognizing that some meanings are tacit in their implicitness as they are embedded yet unspoken in text. In studying the subjectivities of the newborn we need to constantly question the language we use in our interpretations because language itself shapes our primal perception of experience. As Gadamer (2004) writes, "All understanding is interpretation, and all interpretation takes place in the medium of a language that allows the object to come into words and yet is at the same time the interpreter's own language" (p. 390).

A discussion of lived experience should alert us to the primality of existence we experience in the presence of the baby's wandering gaze, as we watch the baby shudder before stilling. The image evoked in the description of the newborn lets us understand something, even though we may not know what this is or struggle to use words to describe it. We experience that a lived experience exists in the presence of a newborn whose look confirms a being here. Yet, we may wonder how such being differs from that of the adult. We need to consider what language we use to convey a sense of the lived experience of a newborn.

What Kind of Consciousness is Composed in a Newborn's Existence?

In an adjacent isolette, a newborn receives analgesic, sedative, and paralytic medications as we struggle to maintain oxygenation. The baby lies splayed. Only the chest moves, vibrating in response to the airflow of the oscillation machine. With muscles relaxed, she cannot move, let alone open her eyes. As we are talking next to the isolette, the baby's heart rate rises.

When watching this baby we cannot help but wonder, does this baby experience anything? Does she feel pain or discomfort, isolation or loneliness? Is she somehow aware of our presence? If our spoken words have an effect on the physiology of her heart rate, does that mean that they also affect her mind? And if so, would that be a sign of conscious awareness?

Consciousness refers to the awareness of our existence of being-in-the-world. It describes a state or condition of sentience—a capacity to feel, perceive, experience. The term 'consciousness' also implies self-awareness—a capacity to distinguish self from world. But we need to make a further distinction between a condition of sentient self-awareness and reflective self-awareness. We speak of someone being conscious as being responsively aware of objects and people around him or her; and, we also speak of being conscious as being self-aware whereby a subject is aware of his or her own subjectivity.

From a phenomenological perspective, consciousness is allied to the notion of lived experience as the "intrinsic feature" of the way we find ourselves experiencing the world as a subject (Zahavi, 2005, p. 20). Consciousness occurs by way of our direct perception of the world. Husserl (1991) describes this primordial awareness as a primal impressional consciousness—a kind of proto-consciousness structured like a temporal streaming 'now-awareness,' that includes a sense of the retentional 'just-now' and the protentional 'next-now' (p. 50). Such a structure of consciousness would seem to be needed to hear music as a melody compared to a series of tones without coherence: a capacity of which a newborn appears capable, emerging in likely a rudimentary form as early as 28 weeks gestation (Draganova et al., 2007; Holst et al., 2005). Primal does not mean unconscious but preconscious. Preconsciousness is already a form of consciousness. At this level we should assume that a newborn is indeed infused with primal or preconscious consciousness such that a preconscious awareness is not (or not yet) reflectively aware of itself.

A phenomenological understanding of consciousness does not eclipse the meaning of the unconscious. It is not that we carry out our activities unconsciously but rather that we tend to be immersed, absorbed, engaged, and preoccupied by objects, events, and other happenings in our subjective day-to-day existence. Even if lived experience is not explicitly conscious, we do live in a context of anticipation. We slide from one encounter into another, and one experience sinks into the other, and indeed in such a way that we do not bother about it. We are immersed in the temporally particular situation and in the unbroken succession of situations that we live through. We are engrossed in it; we do not view ourselves or bring ourselves to a meditative, deliberative, or reflective consciousness as now this comes along or now that (Heidegger, 1962, p. 92).

Subjectivity as related to conscious self-awareness has long been a concern of phenomenology, as witnessed in the classic writings of Husserl, Heidegger, Sartre, and Merleau-Ponty and in the recent writings of Marion, Nancy, Malabou, and Zahavi. It is not enough to say that phenomenology regards things from a first-person point-of-view because this is true of many other qualitative research methodologies such as narrative inquiry, social constructivism, and perception studies. Rather, for phenomenology subjectivity is bound up with lived experience "because the subject that I am, when taken concretely, is inseparable from this body and this world" (Merleau-Ponty, 1962, p. 475).

Lived experience is subjective in that each conscious experience we have appears as our own—as *my experience*. It is not that phenomenology posits that conceptually a *self* exists but that our conscious experience of the world is implicitly marked by "first-personal givenness" to myself as a subject (Zahavi, 2005, p. 22). It is the sensibility that, when I have an experience (something happens to me, or I perceive something) that I am primordially aware that this is my experience and not someone else's. However, this awareness is only primordially mine—I *know* that I *am* this experience. For example, this pain is me. Pain is not some-thing that I possess like an object. Rather this pain is my subjectivity. We may see evidence for such a sensibility in the infant who responds to self-touch differently than the other-touch of an object or other subject (Butterworth & Hopkins, 1988; Rochat & Hespos, 1997; Rochat et al., 1988) such that we may speculate that even from early gestation there is a primal dimension to our awareness of self as *same*, rather than *other*, even if such distinctions are incomplete or emergent.

For the newborn, the world presents itself as a bodily being-in-the-world. Rochat (2001) describes this as our "embodied self" whereby the newborn world consists of direct and immediate perception, contrasting it with "intentional self": the self-conscious reflective awareness of one's "own body as a differentiated entity in the environment" (p. 76). Rochat postulates the self as embodied to develop from as early as within the womb while the self as intentional subject only begins to emerge around the second month of life. In other words, it is only with time that infants are able to "bypass the immediacy of perception to start reflecting on it" (p. 180). I do note to the reader that Rochat's use of the word intentional differs from the notion of *intentionality* as used in the phenomenological literature.

From the work of Rochat and others it may be tempting to believe that different kinds of consciousness exist, or that it is only when consciousness meets a particular level of development that meaning is possible. Yet, if meaning is ultimately founded in the manner in which we live through the world in the immediacy of perception, it is hard not to assume that the consciousness of the newborn is meaningful.

The notion of newborn subjectivity is only problematic if we consider the *self* as a phenomenally distinct, unitary, or pure entity existing over and above our stream of conscious experience. If not, how could we know whether a contemplative self truly exists. Instead, we need to consider subjectivity as existential in its corporeal, spatial, temporal, material, and relational being. Still, for the newborn, are distinctions between self and the world so clear? May we not assume that the responsiveness that we observe in a newborn's heart rate to a heard voice already corresponds to a conscious experience? Is it not likely that subjectivity as self-awareness is always, already present in a most basic primordial sense?

Yet, consciousness in the newborn is enigmatic in that a newborn's bodily perceptual abilities differ from that of an adult. It is not simply that a newborn has different capacities of vision, hearing, smell, and touch; but also that these sense experiences may possess (amodal or multimodal) textures that transcend any single sensory modality (Johnson, 2007; Stern, 1985). The challenge of understanding the nature of the lived experience of this passively quiescent newborn is that we must acknowledge that it may radically differ from our own. The newborn's existence may be marked by relatively undifferentiated temporal contours of pace, rhythm, and intensity. For example, for the newborn the voice that whispers in repetition "Shhhh, Shhhh, Shhhh" may be experientially fused with the hand that touches "Pat, Pat, Pat."

This realization of the unique nature of newborn experience does not need to leave phenomenological research of the newborn at an impasse. Rather, we are brought to wonder about the meaning and significance of primal consciousness when watching the newborn's behavior. Consider for example the infant who cries when someone leaves the room. While we do not know whether such an experience makes an infant feel sad, pained, or angry, we might wonder, for example, whether the cry expresses more fundamentally an "impression of incompleteness" (Merleau-Ponty, 2007, p. 153). This does not mean that the infant truly perceives others as distinct beings compared to him or herself, but rather that the child's cry expresses a primal sense of lack, such that the child's being is experienced as incomplete—yet simultaneously completing in response to the presence of others. So, while the emotionality and psychological meaning of such experiences are perhaps unknowable, we may still gain understandings as to the plausible meaningfulness of such experiences. The enigma of the newborn experience calls for a phenomenology of the meaning of newborn subjectivity, presence, the self, and consciousness.

To conclude, an inquiry into newborn consciousness should alert us to the primordiality of existence when we observe how the infant's heart rate rises in response to a voice. Even though we do not know exactly what constitutes the infant's awareness of his or her world, we experience that the infant, even while being unable to move, is still responsive to the voices around him or her. We sense the existence of a consciousness even if it is enigmatic for us in its subjectivity. The question of the meaning and beginning of consciousness is just as enigmatic as the question of the beginning of life. Heidegger (2012) spoke of inceptuality of meaning as the "thinking out of the beginning" (p. 46). There is no prior question possible for the inceptuality of life and consciousness. It is significant that the phenomenology of neonatology has a unique womb-world concern with the beginning of life and consciousness: it is in the life of the newborn where inceptuality finds the beginning of its beginning.

Do Newborns Live in Their Own World?

> Our first baby was very colicky which was exhausting to say the least. I remember going through the motions of trying to keep him settled and calm. Holding him, rocking him, doing all manners of things so he would just settle. I remember of course being worried about him as much as being worried about my wife. We were exhausted. Then one day it happened, I was changing his diaper when suddenly he looked at me and smiled. I was caught in his gaze.

Are newborn babies capable of eye contact? If not, when does it first occur? What is the meaningfulness of this experience for the parent? But even more puzzling, what might the newborn baby experience? What insights do we have into the intersubjectivity of contact in the newborn's early life experience?

Intersubjectivity is a major topic in phenomenology concerned with the experience of a shared world. It is problematic to view any individual as existing wholly in a private world, whereby the meaning that constitutes his or her existence is defined apart from other individuals. Intersubjectivity after all is a necessary requisite for empathy, play, conversation, and other social experiences.

Some physicians explain that since a newborn's visual acuity is quite coarse, he or she certainly cannot look an other in the eye because the world is simply blurry to them. Others say that, yes, a baby can look at you, a baby can fixate on you, but it is not quite looking you in the eye. Instead a baby looks at you much like at any other thing in the world such as a mobile, a soother, or other object within his or her field of view.

But there is some moment, often around two months of age, when a parent really senses the *look* of a baby: "You can see them look at you! And you appreciate being seen." Perhaps the baby smiles or frowns with such looks. Is it a look of contact, recognition? Is this look betraying an inner awareness of your attentiveness? Perhaps the baby is playing with you during such looks? It seems clear that this *look* is quite different from the earlier newborn stare.

In being seen by the sudden eye contact with the infant we seem to experience the interiority of this child. We may question what we failed to see or perhaps even what we saw in moments before. We may not explicitly realize that the eye contact is a real meeting with a developing consciousness, but that is where phenomenological reflection must do its interpretive work.

Although we need to recognize that the world of the newborn differs from the world of the older child at two months of age or beyond, we still need to question the possible meaningfulness of a newborn existence. Regardless as to whether newborns exist in a contemplative world, do meanings not inceptually inhere within? What meanings exist and evolve in calm or crying states? What meanings lie between? Rochat plays down the significance of the sense of real contact that the infant look may suggest.

> The neonatal world is not a contemplative or conversational world, even if it might seem so to caregivers when they have prolonged eye contacts with newborns. In such stances, newborns often seem to look through you with a flat affect, and often end up closing their eyes and falling asleep. When smiling, usually it is with the eyes closed or semiclosed in the bliss of satiety that follows feeding. They express comfort and well-being, but in essence, they do so involuntarily. In a world that oscillates between slow motion in a calm state and tense agitation in a crying state, newborns perceive and act

directly, with no room for reflection and conscious simulation of what is going to happen next.

(Rochat, 2001, pp. 178–179)

But how is this contact in the intersubjective neonatal world experienced by the parent?

In everyday life, we often interact with newborns as if they have the capacity to understand us and as if they experience the world similar to us. We counter-factually seem to assume that a newborn is able to understand what he or she is not yet able to acknowledge. This *not yet* is the pedagogical trust in the child's developmental promise. Almost from birth, parents and other caregivers interact with young children in a manner that differs from other human relations: they constantly presume abilities and behaviors in the child (such as language and intentionalities) as if they are already present but that still need to be realized. For example, a mother may engage her child in motherese speech as if the child already possesses language competence; or a father may interpret a child's crying in a manner (for example, as being hungry, in pain, annoyed, frightened) as if the child intended this interpretation. But the point is that there is a sense of peda-gogical relationality in the encounter between parent and child. For the parent, the caring adult–infant relation is a relation *sui generis*, which means that the pedagogical quality of this relation is unique and resists being reduced to other human relations (Spiecker, 1984).

There is not always a presumed congruency though between the worlds of the newborn and the adult. When, as physicians, nurses, and caregivers we encounter others in our day-to-day life, we rarely wonder whether these others apprehend the world differently. Of course, there are moments when intersubjective assumptions and understandings have the potential to break down: when a phy-sician is confronted by a patient experiencing hallucinations; when a nurse tends to a patient in the late stages of Alzheimer's disease; or, when a parent tries to calm their colicky newborn. In such situations, we may wonder what this other person is experiencing. This is perhaps all the more the case in a NICU where different medications and technologies are utilized for treatment. At times, parents can be quite confused about what is going on with their newborn.

At other times, health professionals and parents may find themselves intuitively perceiving, feeling, or sensing the meaningfulness apparent in a patient's beha-viors. The physician sees the hallucinating patient responding to perceptions even if such perceptions lack a basis in reality; the nurse may be touched by the dis-orientation of Alzheimer's even if she may not know what has been forgotten; and, parents may hear the unrest in the cry of their colicky newborn even if they do not understand the inner meaning of this unrest. It is not that we project our own experiential sense on the behavior of an other so much that we gain an empathic understanding that is more direct, immediate, corporeal, and perhaps truly primordial.

Merleau-Ponty (1962) says, "we have no right to level all experiences down to a single world, all modalities of existence down to a single consciousness" (p. 338). For human science inquiry into the experiential life of the newborn, the task for phenomenology is to explore the meanings of *possible* different modalities of experience without simply reducing such experiences to our own. In other words, intersubjectivity cannot be reduced to subjectivity.

What Does It Mean to Understand a Newborn's World?

Tucked in at the end of the row, a premature baby seems almost too well to be in intensive care. A nurse brings a soother towards his mouth. He puckers his lower lip and rolls his tongue. Stroking the soother against the corner of his mouth, the nurse pauses for a brief moment. The baby's eyes are fixed firmly on her. Taking the soother in, he gives it a few short sucks before letting it fall off to the side.

How does a newborn experience the presence of others? How does this baby's mouth experience the soother thing? What does he perceive in the face of the nurse? What meaning constitutes his existence?

Meaning is a complex and complicated notion in phenomenology. Phenomenological meaning relates to experiential meanings as they arise in human existence. It is therefore not enough to speak conceptually about an experience as composed of sadness, angst, anxiety, worry, joy, or any other emotion or psychological reaction. Rather, concern is directed at how an experience is lived through which makes it possible to use such emotive terms to begin with.

It is precisely because phenomenological research seeks to explore, understand, and articulate experiences in their lived throughness that as a method it is suited for inquiry into the existence of the newborn. While we cannot know whether our emotive language appropriately names and describes fetal and newborn experiences, we may still use language to wonder about the meanings that give rise to such experiences in their meaningfulness. In the effort to focus on lived experience, phenomenology aims to return to experience in its immediacy for contemplative reflection. But both our understanding of own experiences and our understanding of other people's experiences are always limited for reasons of temporality and relationality.

The French philosopher Levinas (1969) has pointed out that the persons we live with or encounter in our social relations can never be truly understood in their otherness. We always tend to reduce the person we meet to our own impressions and interests—in other words to our self. Ultimately the otherness of the other remains a mystery to us. Many parents have experienced this realization in a moment of awe and wonder, when they gaze at their child and suddenly realize how this little person who they seem to know so well is really a stranger.

This is what Levinas talks about as being addressed by the otherness of the other. In such a moment, I do not encounter the other as a self who is in a mutual relation with me as a self. Rather, I pass over myself and meet the other in his or her true otherness, an otherness that is irreducible to me or to my own interests in the world (Levinas, 1969, pp. 187–253). Especially when we feel addressed by the vulnerability of the premature or ill newborn we experience our response to this vulnerability as response-ability. What happens is that this child has made an appeal on me already. I cannot help but feel responsible even before I may want to feel responsible.

So, on the one hand, we cannot really approach the newborn from any other perspective than our own. No matter how abstract or highly theoretical our scientific research into the perceptional experiences of the newborn might be, it is nevertheless the case that an adult's experience is the necessary point of departure. On the other hand, we can be sensitive to the enigma of the otherness of the newborn. This sensitivity can serve as a gradual awakening to and a constant reminder of the similar-but-different modes of being of the newborn. According to Levinas (1969) this sensitivity is always necessarily ethical. Our attempt at understanding the nature and content of consciousness and subjective experience of the newborn confirms the ethical essence of the relation in which we stand to this newborn person.

And to What Evidence Do We Turn?

The above examples and reflections may suggest that phenomenological studies of the subjectivities and inner lives of newborn babies have to depend on speculative reflection. However, speculation is practiced with respect to matters about which we can prove to be correct or incorrect, at some point in the inquiry. We may speculate that a certain intervention or medication reduces the risks of infection, and subsequently discover that our speculation was correct or incorrect. But insights into the nature of the experience of a newborn cannot be produced through speculation. We may never know whether our description of a newborn's existence is correct or incorrect. In fact, it is not a matter of correctness but of understanding.

Even in adult–adult relations empathic understanding is to be distinguished from factual correctness. How confident can we be that descriptions of adult experiences are correct? Phenomenological researchers frequently employ interview, observation, writing, and other empirical practices to gather material for the crafting of phenomenological human science texts. Concrete accounts of experiences in the form of anecdotes, narratives, or stories have been referred to as 'lived experience descriptions' (van Manen, 1990, 2014). Although these experiential descriptions are starting points for reflection, the experiences in themselves are always unique and singular. Phenomenology explores a manifold of recognizable experiences in order to gain insights into human phenomena that may be evoked by them (van Manen, 2014).

The notion of 'bracketing' originated in the phenomenological tradition as a method of 'unmediated seeing' (*das unmittelbare sehen*)—to place in abeyance assumptions, constructions, and other perspectives so that the focus is the experience as it is actually lived through (Husserl, 1989, p. 54). Some researchers in the human sciences have conceptualized bracketing as a method to mitigate bias so the researcher is essentially free of assumptions, values, interests, theories, and so forth. But that is a misunderstanding. One cannot free oneself of the knowledge that constitutes the pre-understandings one has of the world anymore than one can free oneself of being-in-the-world. Nor does there exist a singular, true, objective understanding of the world. Even objectivity has its own subjectivity. And yet, one may be able to become aware of pre-understandings and how they play a role in our lived world.

Merleau-Ponty (1964b) argues that the philosopher "is not disqualified to reinterpret facts he has not observed himself, if these facts say something more and different than what the scientist has seen in them" (p. 101). So, the question is, what empirical data are appropriate to stir reflection on a particular lived experience? We may use the term *constatation* to refer to a reflective understanding of an empirical statement that can be employed for phenomenological inquiry and show by example such an approach. Linquistically, a *constative* is a speech act: "a statement that is capable of being true or false" (*OED*). Constatations are the reflective results of constating. In the context of phenomenology, the purpose of the constatation is to explore experiential meanings. Constative reflection is the attempt at phenomenal truth by exploring the meaningfulness of an experience that is based on established empirical evidence.

For example, a well-known empirical study by DeCasper and Fifer (1980) bears the title "Of Human Bonding: Newborns Prefer Their Mothers' Voices."

> By sucking a nonnutritive nipple in different ways, a newborn human could produce either its mother's voice or the voice of another female. Infants learned how to produce the mother's voice and produced it more often than the other voice.
>
> (DeCasper & Fifer, 1980, p. 1174)

The primary conclusion from this study was that newborns "demonstrate a preference for their mothers' voices" (DeCasper & Fifer, 1980, p. 1176). Yet the empirical finding of newborns' differentially sucking in response to their mothers' voice can be variably interpreted and questioned. Is 'preference' the correct word to describe the subjectivity experienced by a newborn? How do newborns actually experience 'fondness or partiality' as conceptualized in these studies? Experimental observations may lead us to wonder whether newborns have primal experiences of 'familiarity,' but what would these experiences of preference, fondness, or partiality consist in? What words evoke the phenomenological experiential meanings?

When we consider all of the recent research showing differential responses of newborn infants to their mother's voice, smell, taste, and other sense material, perhaps the basic insight is more simply that newborns are actually not new to the world—the mother's voice is a known voice to the newborn. But that still leaves in abeyance the question of the phenomenality of the meaning of these new-borns' experiences. Might the primary constatation be that the newborn recog-nizes the mother's voice in the above research example? The term 'preference' connotes a greater liking of one alternative above another (*OED*), but is that what the newborn experiences? Is it a matter of alternative choices that the research uncovers? Or is it more accurately a sense of familiarity that draws the infant? Next we might ask, what is the sensuality of this sense of familiarity that is explained as a 'demonstration of preference' by the researcher?

Findings of empirical studies can be useful to the phenomenological researcher provided the researcher is prepared to question the ontological presumptions that belong to the language of the scientific discipline. Psychology has developed such phrases as 'preference behaviors' and 'habituation behaviors' to describe the activities that newborns engage in during such experiments. A certain intuition of what constitutes an object, activity, or being is always already implied in experi-mental investigation. Put differently, "for every assertion of experimental psy-chology a corresponding eidetic assertion can be found" (Merleau-Ponty, 1964b, pp. 72, 73). As phenomenologists, we need to return to the experiential dimen-sions of the experiments themselves rather than rely on the language of the experimental synopsis if we are going to endeavor to explore the possibilities of using empirical research for constative phenomenological reflection on the lived meaning of these findings.

Phenomenology as a search and exploration for the meanings inherent in lived experience does not need to occur apart from insights from empirical studies. And in turn, empirical sciences may benefit from phenomenological inquiries to point to possibilities of experiential understanding.

> A science without philosophy would literally not know what it was talking about. A philosophy without methodical exploration of phenomena would end up with nothing but formal truths, which is to say, errors.
>
> *(Merleau-Ponty, 1964c, p. 97)*

Engaging with empirical research offers many potential benefits. For example, connecting phenomenological reflection with empirical studies may demonstrate the contemporary relevance of phenomenology. Constatations may also invite and challenge the personal viewpoints of researchers or simply challenge phe-nomenological questions. Still, the phenomenological researcher needs to be able to put claims made by the empirical sciences aside in order to make room for an investigation of the meanings of lived experience. Some space needs to be pre-served between phenomenology and the empirical sciences such that the aim of phenomenological research is to arrive at the lived meanings of these constative reflections.

References

Butterworth, G., & Hopkins, B. (1988). "Hand-mouth coordination in the new-born baby." *British Journal of Developmental Psychology*, 6(4), 303–314.

DeCasper, A. J., & Fifer, W. P. (1980). "Of human bonding: newborns prefer their mothers' voices." *Science*, 208(4448), 1174–1176.

Draganova, R., Eswaran, H., Murphy, P., Lowery, C., & Preissl, H. (2007). "Serial magnetoencephalographic study of fetal newborn auditory discriminative evoked responses." *Early Human Development*, 83(3), 199–207.

Gadamer, H.-G. (2004). *Truth and Method*. (J. Weinsheimer, D. G. Marshall, transl.) London: Continuum. (Original work published 1975).

Heidegger, M. (1962). *Being and Time*. (J. Macquarrie, E. Robinson, transl.) New York, NY: Harper & Row. (Original work published 1927).

Heidegger, M. (2012). *Contributions to Philosophy (of the Event)*. (R. Rojcewicz, D. Vallega-Neu, transl.) Bloomington, IN: Indiana University Press. (Original work published 1989).

Holst, M., Eswaran, H., Lowery, C., Murphy, P., Norton, J., & Preissl, H. (2005). "Development of auditory evoked fields in human fetuses newborns: a longitudinal MEG study." *Clinical Neurophysiology*, 116(8), 1949–1955.

Husserl, E. (1989). *Ideas Pertaining to a Pure Phenomenology and to a Phenomenological Philosophy. Second Book: General Introduction to a Pure Phenomenology*. (R. Rojcewicz, A. Schuwer, transl.) Dordrecht: Kluwer. (Original work published 1913).

Husserl, E. (1991). *On the Phenomenology of the Consciousness of Internal Time (1893–1917)*. (J. B. Brough, transl.) Dordrecht: Kluwer Academic. (Original work published 1966).

James, W. (1890). *Principles of Psychology*. New York, NY: Henry Holt and Company.

Johnson, M. (2007). *The Meaning of the Body: Aesthetics of Human Understanding*. Chicago, IL: University of Chicago Press.

Levinas, E. (1969). *Totality and Infinity: An Essay on Exteriority*. (A. Lingis, transl.) Pittsburgh, PA: Duquesne University Press. (Original work published 1961).

Marlier, L., & Schaal, B. (2005). "Human newborns prefer human milk: conspecific milk odor is attractive without postnatal exposure." *Child Development*, 76(1), 155–168.

Marlier, L., Gaugler, C., Astruc, D., & Messer, J. (2007). "La sensibilité olfactive du nouveau-né prématuré" [The olfactory sensitivity of the premature newborn]. *Archives De Pédiatrie, 14*(1), 45–53.

Merleau-Ponty, M. (1962). *Phenomenology of Perception*. (C. Smith, transl.) London: Routledge & Kegan Paul Ltd. (Original work published 1945).

Merleau-Ponty, M. (1964a). "Phenomenology and the sciences of man." (J. Wild, transl.) In: J. M. Edie (ed.), *The Primacy of Perception and Other Essays on Phenomenological Psychology, the Philosophy of Art, History and Politics*. Evanston, IL: Northwestern University Press. pp. 43–95. (Original work published 1961).

Merleau-Ponty, M. (1964b). *Signs*. (R. C. McCleary, transl.) Evanston, IL: Northwestern University Press. (Original work published 1960).

Merleau-Ponty, M. (1964c). *Sense and Non-Sense*. (H. L. Dreyfus, P. A. Dreyfus, transl.) Evanston, IL: Northwestern University Press. (Original work published 1948).

Merleau-Ponty, M. (2007). "The child's relations with others." (J. Wild, transl.) In: T. Toadvine & L. Lawlor (eds.), *The Merleau-Ponty Reader*. Evanston, IL: Northwestern University Press. pp. 143–183. (Original work published 1951).

Ricoeur, P. (1966). *Freedom and Nature: The Voluntary and the Involuntary*. (E. V. Kohák, Trans.). Evanston, IL: Northwestern University Press. (Original work published 1950).

Rochat, P. (2001). *The Infant's World*. Cambridge, MA: Harvard University Press.

Rochat, P., & Hespos, S. J. (1997). "Differential rooting response by neonates: evidence for an early sense of self." *Early Development and Parenting*, 6(3–4), 105–112.

Rochat, P., Blass, M., & Hoffmeyer, L. B. (1988). "Oropharyngeal control of hand-mouth coordination in newborn infants." *Developmental Psychology*, 24(4), 459–463.

Romano, C. (2015). *At the Heart of Reason*. (M. B. Smith, C. Romano, transl.) Evanston, IL: Northwestern University Press. (Original work published 2010).

Spiecker, B. (1984). "The pedagogical relationship." *Oxford Review of Education*, 10(2), 203–209.

Stern, D. N. (1985). *The Interpersonal World of the Infant: A View from Psychoanalysis and Developmental Psychology*. New York, NY: Basic Books.

Van Manen, M. (1990). *Researching Lived Experience: Human Science for an Action Sensitive Pedagogy*. Albany, NY: SUNY Press; London, ON: Althouse Press.

Van Manen, M. (2014). *Phenomenology of Practice: Meaning-Giving Methods in Phenomenological Research and Writing*. Walnut Creek, CA: Left Coast Press.

Waldenfels, B. (2007). *The Question of the Other*. Hong Kong: The Chinese University Press.

Zahavi, D. (2005). *Subjectivity and Selfhood: Investigating the First-Person Perspective*. Cambridge, MA: MIT Press.

2

WITHIN THE WOMB WORLD

[The house] is the human being's first world. Before he is "cast into the world," ... man is laid in the cradle of the house. And always, in our daydreams, the house is a large cradle ... Life begins well, it begins enclosed, protected, all warm in the bosom of the house.

(Bachelard, 1994, p. 5)

In his *Poetics of Space*, Gaston Bachelard explores the images of our primal dwelling: the house and its rooms, corners, crannies, and the forgotten things of our existence that still silently live within us. He points out that our soul is an abode too. And by remembering our first home, we learn to abide within ourselves. The images are as much in us as we are in them. The house as our first and primal abode offers shelter and protection, and, says Bachelard, "whenever the human being has found the slightest shelter: we shall see the imagination build 'walls' of impalpable shadows, comfort itself with the illusion of protection—or, just the contrary, tremble behind thick walls" (p. 5). The image of the house and its walls harbor within themselves the meaning and significance of the cradle of our existence. Our house is the shell in which we know ourselves sheltered and to which we must return in our waking and nocturnal dreams.

But more primordial even than the image of the house and cradle is the maternal womb in which life finds its first stirrings. What is our image of this original cradle where life itself finds its wondrous inception? And what interior images are laid down in the fetal beings who find in the womb their source and inceptuality of their existence as singular beings? Like the protective walls of the house, the maternal body houses a walled womb. *Wombe, wambe,* and *wambō* name the mother's belly, stomach, or abdomen. These are the outer walls that shelter the fetus, the growing child within. I propose that we need to trace

Bachelard's primal image of the cradle even further back to the womb, and ask how understanding the womb helps us appreciate the world of the newborn. More so, constative reflecting on the phenomenology of the womb raises questions for the pedagogy of neonatal intensive care where a more technological image of the cradle becomes the substitute for the primordial image of the womb. What are some of the present and latent implications of that substitution?

Some scientific literature conceives of the mother's belly as an insulating space for wombed being whereby the condition of the fetus is sometimes conceived in terms of images of unconscious sleep, indeterminate sleep, and transitionings between such sleep stages (Lagercrantz & Changeux, 2009; Mellor et al., 2005). But the assumption that the fetus exists in a state of unconsciousness is problematic. Extensive fetal behavior literature reveals that the womb is a place of sensate existence, and that it is formative of activities, perceptions, and memories (Platt, 2011). Of course, speculations regarding the sensuality of womb need to be cautiously tempered by the realization of the limits and lack of our understanding as to whether the fetus has the capacity for sensations resembling more mature conscious or preconscious experiences. Does the fetus exist in some states of conscious awareness or even rudimentary forms of preconsciousness? And if indeed fetal consciousness exists, how is it fundamentally comparable, and perhaps similar or dissimilar to the conscious awareness, sub-awareness, or pre-reflexive awareness of the newborn, older child, or adult?

The womb is the inceptual place of conception, where the self finds its beginning. This 'embryonic' or 'incipient' self of the wombed fetal child should not be confused with a reflective or self-conscious self. We cannot yet speak of a proper or developed self that dwells within the womb: the fetal child as a prenatal human is coming-into-being as a being connected, within, and part of its mother. *Fetus* means offspring, bringing forth (*OED*). To use the term 'fetus,' by thus likening the fetal child to the premature child, is existentially inappropriate as it implies a separate coming-into-being. Instead, the fetal body is in-complete, a plurality of developing senses, only intelligible when understood as composed of sensuality in-uterus or in-wombed.

Despite the obvious limitations that constrain our experiential understanding of the womb world, we may still constatively reflect on the possible sense and sensuality of the womb for the womb-child, the existential traces of which we recognize when a newborn calms in response to being held and swaddled; when a newborn stills in response to his or her mother's heartbeat; or, when a newborn startles in the presence of a bright light. How does experiential human life begin within another human being? What are the conditions and paths of becoming for the fetus within the womb?

First Contact

Embryology tells the story of a cell becoming clusters of cells that develop and differentiate, from cleavage and compaction, sulcation and folding, to become the bodily tissue that we name the 'fetus' at nine weeks gestation (Sadler, 2015). Discernible movements appear between seven and eight-and-a-half weeks gestation, with responsiveness to touch following (de Vries et al., 1982). Scientific evidence suggests the possibility, if not probability, that the capacity for perception in some form emerges some time around 20 weeks gestation (Platt, 2011). The fetal tissues gradually form into a singularity, though the fetus or wombed child remains singular in plurality well until birth—interconnected with the maternal body.

The fetal sense and sensuality of the womb seem to have a presence without a determinable beginning. It is the beginning and unfolding of life itself. The temperature of the amniotic fluid bathing the fetus is almost constant in temperature, slowly fluctuating only by fractions of a degree throughout the day in response to changes in maternal temperature (Asakura, 2004). Always having been bathed in warm amniotic fluid, the constatation is that sensuality is ceaseless. We may wonder if the sensuality of warmth is even felt when its absence or opposite, cold, has not yet occurred. Ever present and without variation, sensuality seems contingent on that which is yet to come. For example, disruption of this constancy by means of artificially cooling the amniotic fluid of a pregnant animal in an experimental setting, elicits arousal and activity in the fetus (Schwab et al., 1997). So it appears that sensory recognition requires divergence. Does the sensation of warmth emerge alongside the capacity for temperature sensation against a background of insensate nihility? Or perhaps, does lack of warmth only become felt once the infant is born into a cold world?

Without unmethodically committing to the premise that sense is experienced as meaningful for the fetus, we may constatively reflect that sensuality is laden with meaning in its contingency. In a raw sense, the sensuality of the womb consists in part of a kind of perception that bears the smell and taste of the mother: the amniotic fluid literally is of her flavor (Mennella, 2007). Even before the capacity to suck and swallow develops, olfaction is present in at least a rudimentary form as early as 20 weeks gestation (Schaal et al., 2004). From a constatative meaning perspective, we see traces of this sensuality as the newborn child seems drawn to the unique scent of the mother and the taste of her breast milk (Bartocci et al., 2000; Marlier et al., 1998). It seems that a sensuality of constancy makes sense in its eventuality, establishing the possibility of familiarity in a fundamental manner. And of course, tastes and smells evoke different responses: to the taste of sweetness, newborns smile, suck, and lick; and, to sour taste, newborns purse their lips, wrinkle their noise, and blink (Soussignan et al., 1997).

More philosophically, birth dis-embodies the embodied. Birth detaches and removes a newborn from what had constituted its sense-existence as a fetus. To seek and orient to the mother's milk is to re-appropriate and re-embody what was lost. When the newborn is placed against his or her mother's breasts and stomach, the mother's body becomes an external womb. We wonder: does the phenomenon of birth, de-wombing, leave the newborn incomplete and therefore with a lack, and therefore with the capacity for embodiment? In other words, does an inceptual beginning of a bodily being with an other leave the newborn expectant for the presence of others.

Amniotic fluid gives buoyancy and resistance to the fetal singularity. And as pregnancy progresses, the growing fetal body increasingly 'meets' the enclosing uterine walls. Movement is contained such that to the observer of a prenatal ultrasound image the womb world appears as a holding place. From a medical perspective, we know that holding in a free manner is crucial for development. Pregnancies complicated by lack of amniotic fluid (anhydramnios) result in joint contractures, because the fetus has been held unable to move. The extreme situation is Potter (1946) sequence, the classic chain of events resulting from lack of kidney development (bilateral renal agenesis). Without sufficient fluid, the maternal uterus compresses, physically deforming the face, skull, and limbs. In the womb world, holding is not restraint. Even in the final weeks of pregnancy, when the fetus is closely contained, arms, hands, trunk, and legs can move despite being held in fluid flexion.

The constation is that the capacity for movement, even if contained, suggests that sensuality has margins, barriers, and limits. Of course, it is not clear whether the fetal body senses such limits as external to its body; or whether such points of contact are sensually not contacts at all, but instead a corporeally entwined bodily being in itself whereby the maternal body is not separate from the fetal form. Merleau-Ponty (2007) uses the word *syncretic* to describe such a state of being: "there is not one individual over against another but rather an anonymous collectivity, an undifferentiated group life" (p. 149). So, when the infant calms to being held or swaddled, or when the baby calms to external presence, this may be sensed as a pressure of familiarity, a fetal way of being-in-the-womb-world.

Ultrasound observers have described a complex repertoire of movements of the fetus joined to that of the mother's body (de Vries et al., 1985). The fetal singularity reacts to its mother's actions, bouncing up and down with her laughter. Even the simple act of walking may cause the fetus to swivel or rock. In other words, there are constatative dimensions to the kinetic sensuality of the womb. Perception is provoked by the changing contact of the fetus with the uterine wall and the emerging capacities of the sensory structures. Mothers often report, and ultrasound studies give evidence, that the activity of the fetus varies with the time of day: movements are more common during the night (de Vries et al., 1987). Daytime motion may be sensed as lulling or soothing. And the quietness of the maternal body at night may reflect a deficiency in sensuality to which the fetus responds with activity.

Rhythms

The womb world is a world of rhythms: regular, repetitive, and recurrent. As the uterus abuts against the abdominal aorta, in proximity of the maternal heart, the womb world is accentuated by the constant cadence of the mother's heartbeat.

Contractions of the maternal bowels and other organ noises produce recurring staccatos of bodily sounds and vibrations. A mother's breathing and walking leads to rhythmic rocking of the fetal body. We know the fetus responds to such sounds and vibrations as evidenced in physiological changes as early as 16 weeks gestation and auditory cortex electrographic activity by 25–27 weeks gestation (Kisilevsky et al., 2003; Wilkinson & Jiang, 2006).

The womb, while sheltered in relative darkness, nonetheless has some trans-parencies and permits light to penetrate through. As with sound and vibration, there is rhythmicity to light: the dark of night, and the varying brightnesses of daytime. The fetal eyes, and corresponding neurocortical tracts, while immature, are in a constant state of development. Corresponding to the opening of eyelids at 26 weeks gestation, the fetus may blink or squint in response to bright light, and by 30 weeks gestation has the capacity to fixate vision on a large object in close proximity (Moore et al., 2015). Such development is dependent on varia-tion in sensation—facilitated by the environmental rhythmicity and the emerging capacities of the fetus. For example, red is the first color to which the newborn responds, presumably because of transillumination of maternal oxygenated hemoglobin in the surrounding tissues that produce red radiance during daytime contrasted with darkness of night within the womb (Clark-Gambelunghe & Clark, 2015).

The constatation is that the sensuality of the womb-child possesses a tempor-ality that does not simply persist but also repeats and reverberates. There are recurring and returning sounds, vibrations, lights, and other sensory phenomena. Rhythm presupposes silence and stillness. Reprises require moments of pause, just as reappearances require fading, vanishing, or loss. Also, to feel rhythm requires the ability to feel difference. For the fetus, even as early as 23 weeks gestation, sudden sounds or vibration may precipitate changes in fetal heart rate, physically move, and even causing the fetus to void (Birnholz & Benacerraf, 1983; Leader et al., 1982; Zimmer et al., 1993). So, while it may be hazardous to assert that the fetus experiences feelings such as being startled, surprised, or frightened; we constatate that the fetus does show responses that have sense meanings.

Thus, it would seem that the sensuality of the womb has a temporality that the fetus recognizes. For example, as early as 23 weeks gestation, fetuses may be observed to respond with movement of the trunk or limbs in response to mechanical vibrations applied to the maternal abdominal wall; and yet, following consecutive applications of such vibrations the fetal response appears to cease (Leader et al., 1982). The constatation is that the irregular may become regular in the wombed world.

The fetus may comparatively turn sensitive to sounds and time—such as the temporal spaces between sounds. Multiple empirical studies have demonstrated that newborns seem to remember particular sounds, melodies, and rhythmic poems from their wombed life (Bauer, 2006; DeCasper et al., 1994; Granier-Deferre et al., 2011). So we may consider the constatation that the temporal sense of such sensuality is not simply reflexively given, raising questions of meaning. What does rhythm carry when a newborn child is observed to cry less and gain more weight when exposed to the rhythmic sounds of heartbeat (Salk, 1973)? Or even when a fetus' heart rate slows to the mother's voice of reading a rhyme (DeCasper et al., 1994)? Are rhythms meaningful for the fetus? How does rhythm begin to make sense?

Together Yet Separate

Physiologically the fetal singularity and the maternal body are of a common substance. Various neurotransmitters, peptides, and endocrine factors circulate the maternal body and also traverse the placenta regulating the fetal tissues (Mellor et al., 2005). For example, maternal adenosine suppresses fetal cerebral activity during stress; presumably decreasing fetal metabolism to save needed energy resources to attenuate neural injury in the event that such stress is accompanied by a decreased fetal brain perfusion (Hunter et al., 2003). Generally, we suspect that the neuromodulatory substances that flow across the placenta do not render the fetus completely insensate, yet do have the capacity to effect fetal neurosensory function.

Much clinical scientific research to date has focused on the cumulative impact of maternal mental health on the developing fetus. Epidemiologists and other researchers have explored how various neuromodulators may affect the psychosocial development of the fetus, linking prenatal stress to cognitive, behavioral, and psychosocial outcomes in childhood and beyond (Charil et al., 2010; Sandman et al., 2012; Yong Ping et al., 2015). It would appear that prenatal psychosocial stress is a complex phenomenon that affects maternal emotions, behavior, and physiology, and may influence the fetus through a myriad of different pathways (Beijers et al., 2014). While most research has focused on physiologic mechanisms, we may wonder whether fetal perception is conditioned by the body of the mother. In moments of stress, does maternal excitement, sadness, or other emotions affect the fetus in a sensual manner?

While maternal tissues, muscles, and fat attenuate, muffle and protect the fetus from the outside world, the womb world is nonetheless intermittently pierced by irregular textures of sound, light, and movement, indeterminate and undefined sensualities. Most prominently, the mother's voice reaches the fetus with seemingly little attenuation precisely because of the bodily cohesion of fetal and maternal corporeal form (Busnel, 1979; Querleu et al., 1989; Smith et al., 1990). Thus, we may constatate that the maternal voice is not 'strange' in its latent significance as the newborn baby orients to and exhibits behaviors to elicit her voice soon after birth (DeCasper & Fifer, 1980; Ockleford et al., 1988). What researchers have deemed 'preference' is not simply for the maternal voice but rather for the filtered, low-keyed maternal timbre as heard from within the womb (Fifer & Moon, 1995). Other voices too may become significant as evidenced by newborns' responses to a father's voice that was heard while in the womb (Lee & Kisilevsky, 2014). The constative question becomes: are these voices appreciated simply because of repeated exposure, or in part because of the interrelation of maternal and fetal intercorporeality?

Research suggests that the wombed child does not only respond to the mother's voice in utero but actually orients to her voice when born (Hepper et al., 1993). More so, it appears that a fetus responds differentially, depending on its own resting state and whether the mother is awake and talking, as compared to when she is resting and silent (Voegtline et al., 2013). We need to constatively reflect whether the sensuality of the womb is a common, shared, or united perceptual field joining mother and fetus? After all, some voices, music, or other noises are appreciated by the mother as significant causing her to pause—her body to listen. As the mother's body quiets, there is the possibility that the embodying maternal body is cultivating and conditioning responsivity in the fetus. Presumably maternal surges of adrenaline and other circulating metabolites may affect the being of the fetus such that sensuality is experienced cohesively. Responsivity possibly is born not simply from consistency but also from a sensual corporeal synchronicity of mother and fetus.

It is not simply that the maternal body affects the fetus, but also that the fetus affects the maternal body. Beyond the changes in body size and shape, active movements, the 'kicking' of a fetus, may cause a mother to pause, sit down, or rest. Even movements that are not felt may stimulate a maternal sympathetic response, demonstrating the bidirectional nature of the maternal–fetal relationship (DiPietro et al., 2004). Such surges of responsivity and interactivity may cause the uterus to tighten its hold, and thus to calm the active fetus.

As we learn more about fetal movements from emerging ultrasound technologies, it appears that some early fetal movements have an intentionality or directedness: touching the face, clasping hands, and grabbing feet (Castiello et al., 2010). Such movements are not simply reflexive but are directed as self-touch or other contact. A sensuality of cohesion is marked not only by responsivity but also receptivity. We may see receptivity when the fetus moves in response to touch of the maternal abdomen (Marx & Nagy, 2015). Such responsivity to relational touch is dynamic: early in pregnancy the fetus moves away from touch, whereas later on the fetus moves toward it (Valman & Pearson, 1980). So, we can only wonder whether the fetus is cultivated to calm, or actually calms in response to a mother's hand laid over the abdomen when she notices the active child? Does the fetus develop a sense of being *at home* in the womb world?

Life Beyond the Walled Womb

As early as at 15 weeks gestation, we may observe the fetus to smile with no one able to see it (Piontelli, 2010). These smiles are described as rudimentary, spontaneous, or non-social without external cause, seeming to occur when the fetus is relatively calm or still (Kawakami & Yanaihara, 2012). Buytendijk (1988) suggests that we should be cautious in our exploring, questioning, and interpreting of the smile of the child:

> when the first smile appears, the child may still function in a state which may not be animalistic but which is, nevertheless, a physiologically closed existence—an existence as yet without an inner life. If this were the case then we could not really compare the crying and smiling of the infant with our adult expressions.
>
> *(Buytendijk, 1988, p. 16)*

While we cannot know whether or how the fetus may be said to have an inner life, or even if such an inner life exists, whether it is similar in nature to the inner life of a young child or an adult, we might constatatively raise some questions. Do these smiles betray a sensuality of recognition of the other? Do they indicate the beginning of a certain reflexivity (unaware awareness), a sensation of self? Does the fetal smile speak to a sensuality of life beginning well?

When comparing the fetus in the womb with the premature infant in the NICU several significant questions arise: The first question of neonatology is how does the beginning of life begin? How is the womb the inceptual cradle of the beginning of life? Michel Henry (2008; 2009) would say that this question can never be answered or understood from an external perspective of medical science. Paradoxically, life is the inceptual beginning of itself. Life finds its beginning in the womb world, but even here, as in the external world, we never see life itself. What we see is the living organism of the living being. But we cannot 'see' life in them. The second question of neonatology asks, how does the journey of life begin for a fetus who prematurely becomes a child in the world? What is the significance of being severed from the sensuality of the womb when born premature? Is there a new transitional 'womb' that cradles the premature child? Can the neonatal isolette be considered a transitional womb? What are the sensual consequences of a 'cradle' composed of medical instruments instead of maternal flesh? Some children spend many months in the NICU, the latent importance of which for their neurodevelopment is increasingly being recognized (Santos et al., 2015).

For the premature newborn, the transition to the neonatal isolette is a profound event. Housed in an incubator or bassinette, the floating in the fluid held in the womb is lost as the infant's containment changes into positioning on the dry bed surface supported by cloth rolls, specialty pillows, or other devices (Madlinger-Lewis et al., 2014). As gravity becomes increasingly present, the wet womb movements become impossible for the preterm child such that he or she is stuck on his or her tummy, back, or side. The caregiver must position and reposition the premature child to avoid deformities of the head and pressure sores inflicted from the material of the medical bed (Vergara & Bigsby, 2004). Rather than being carried in the womb, the infant's existence becomes regulated by repeated assessments, and by servo-controlled temperature and humidity settings. The NICU technology creates a new but different constancy, tempered by the medical tactility of the hospital world.

The rhythm of the NICU is also of a different texture compared to the womb world. Bodily sounds and vibrations are replaced by the regularity and irregularity of respiratory machines potentially approaching dangerous volumes for newborn ears (Surenthiran et al., 2013). Mechanical ventilators, bi-level continuous positive airway pressure (CPAP) machines, nasal noninvasive mechanical ventilation (NIMV), and other means of providing breathing support produce rhythmic fluctuations in sound with the rise and fall of airflow. Other devices deliver straight airflow (low flow, high flow, or simple CPAP) and create a continuous, harsh hush attenuating the world beyond the mask. Day–night rhythmicity may be interrupted when light is needed for evening clinical activities, and darkness is introduced inappropriately during the day (Mirmiran & Ariagno, 2000).

Without the cohesion of the fetal with the maternal body, we wonder whether the world of the NICU still has meaning or becomes meaningless. Background voices and other noises are no longer shared with the mother's body. At sudden moments, a medical hand may poke or prod to insert an intravenous line or obtain blood work. With each shift, new doctors, nurses, respiratory therapists, and other health professionals may be seen, felt, smelled, and heard. Parental presence may become intermittent, adversely affecting the infant's wellbeing (Latva et al., 2004; Reynolds et al., 2013). Even the most dedicated parent cannot be physically in contact with their child continuously when faced with other responsibilities. At times, it may only be the deliverance of breast milk that bears the traces of the mother's presence. Thus, inevitably, the baby becomes conjoint with the medical technologies of intravenous lines and gavage tubes (van Manen, 2012).

The relational ambience of the NICU is perhaps more child-with-technology than child-with-parent, or at the very least child-with-technology-with-parent. Of course, we must be careful not to be too critical when even the world of the healthy newborn becomes saturated with technologies: bassinettes, bottles, soothers, monitors, diapers, mobiles, and so forth. Yet in the NICU such technologies may interfere with the relational contact of parent and child (van Manen, 2012). Moments of maternal touch are interrupted by virtue of the need to reach into the isolette to perform necessary medical procedures or assessments; or indeed by the desire to contain or cradle the child between loving hands. While educated parents may take care to offer slow, pressured touch mimicking the uterine wall; other kinds of gestures now occur that were not possible in the womb world: patting, rubbing, and stroking (Smith, 2012). Parental touch in the NICU perhaps has a greater capacity for intention, purpose, or directedness compared to that of the womb world. The parent may respond to their child's cues with their eyes and ears and with new kinds of touch that are perhaps premature. We are suspecting and learning that even seemingly innocent acts, like clothing the premature child, may have latent consequences for a child's behavior (Durier et al., 2015).

Periodically, babies in the NICU will be held skin-to-skin against a parent's chest in kangaroo care. In the presence of the mother, the experience undoubtedly is marked by sensual traces of the womb world as the child encounters maternal smells, body vibrations, and sounds that may benefit the bond for both child and mother (Bayley, 2015). Parents can be observed to spend hours holding their child surrounded by medical monitors and devices, sometimes with equipment draped over their shoulders. In this paradoxical technologized scenic setting, the parent's body may respond to the child with fluid adjustments in position in response to the child's movements. But such hours of skin-to-skin care represent only a fraction of the infant's NICU days. For some families, engaging in kangaroo time beyond a few days or hours a week may be unachievable goal, given socioeconomic constraints and other parental responsibilities (Seidman et al., 2015).

The design and routines of an NICU impacts the contact between infants and their parents (Baylis et al., 2014). For example, a growing NICU design trend is the movement to single-family rooms rather than open-bay designs (Stevens et al., 2015). The motivation behind this change is to create private spaces for parents to be with their children to afford the development of intimacy between the child and parent (Shahheidari & Homer, 2012). The walls, doors, and other barriers shield out excessive noise, light, and other noxious stimulation. What is striking about the single-family room is that in the absence of the family presence, and often even with the family's presence, the room may be eerily quiet (Liu, 2012). Gone are the voices and other potentially beneficial noises that were reminiscent of the womb world. The sensuality of the environment thus returns to the immediate white-noised machinery and other background, ruptured sounds. Constancy may truly become stale without the meaningful rhythm of parental presence in the child's world as the single-family room becomes isolating for the infant. It is therefore not surprising that some research points to the potential harm of the single-family room environment for NICU infants: adverse changes in brain growth and, in the long term, delays in language acquisition and motor development (Pineda et al., 2014).

Concluding Thoughts

The striking differences between the sensuality of the walled womb world and NICU emerge from a pedagogical concern: how ought we to care for these children who find themselves prematurely severed from the womb? We may wonder how the NICU environment is 'teaching' infants to touch and be touched, hear and be heard, see and be seen? Even without considering all of the noxious pharmakon events in the NICU of medical procedures, we need to ask constatatively what kind of sensuality are we aiming to cultivate in the NICU?

Do we treat newborns like children who should be in the womb? Do we act as if they were born term? Or should we care for them in such a way that is somehow different from both, but more continuous with the existence of the walled womb? We have responsibilities and opportunities to reflect on these concerns and to interact sensibly and sensitively with these babies for weeks, and sometimes months, before they 'ought' to have been born.

And so, we turn to the phenomenological question regarding the life of the newborn child. We ask what is expressed in the first cry that signals that a new and separate life has begun, the transition from wombed world to the life of the worlded world?

References

Asakura, H. (2004). "Fetal and neonatal thermoregulation." *Journal of Nippon Medical School*, 71(6), 360–370.

Bachelard, G. (1994). *The Poetics of Space*. (M. Jolas, transl.) Boston, MA: Beacon Press. (Original work published 1958).

Bartocci, M., Winberg, J., Ruggiero, C., Bergqvist, L. L., Serra, G., & Lagercrantz, H. (2000). "Activation of olfactory cortex in newborn infants after odor stimulation: a functional near-infrared spectroscopy study." *Pediatric Research*, 48(1), 18–23.

Bauer, P. J. (2006). "Constructing a past in infancy: a neuro-developmental account." *Trends in Cognitive Sciences*, 10(4), 175–191.

Bayley, J., Committee on Fetus and Newborn. (2015). "Skin-to-skin care for preterm infants in the neonatal ICU." *Pediatrics*, 136(3), 596–599.

Baylis, R., Ewald, U., Gradin, M., Hedberg Nyqvist, K., Rubertsson, C., & Thernström Blomqvist, Y. (2014). "First-time events between parents and preterm infants are affected by the designs and routines of neonatal intensive care units." *Acta Paediatrica*, 103(10), 1045–1052.

Beijers, R., Buitelaar, J. K., & de Weerth, C. (2014). "Mechanisms underlying the effects of prenatal psychosocial stress on child outcomes: beyond the HPA axis." *European Child & Adolescent Psychiatry*, 23(10), 943–956.

Birnholz, J. C., & Benacerraf, B. R. (1983). "The development of human fetal hearing." *Science*, 222(4623), 516–518.

Busnel, M. (1979). "Intravaginal measurements of the level and acoustic distortion of maternal noises." *Electrodiagnostic-Therapie*, 16(3), 142.

Buytendijk, F. J. J. (1988). "The first smile of the child." *Phenomenology + Pedagogy*, 6(1), 15–24.

Castiello, U., Becchio, C., Zoia, S., Nelini, C., Sartori, L., Blason, L., D'Ottavio, G., Bulgheroni, M., & Gallese, V. (2010). "Wired to be social: the ontogeny of human interaction." *PLOS One*, 5(10), e13199.

Charil, A., Laplante, D. P., Vaillancourt, C., & King, S. (2010). "Prenatal stress and brain development." *Brain Research Reviews*, 65(1), 56–79.

Clark-Gambelunghe, M. B., & Clark, D. A. (2015). "Sensory development." *Pediatric Clinics of North America*, 62(2), 367–384.

De Vries, J. I., Visser, G. H., & Prechtl, H. F. (1982). "The emergence of fetal behaviour: I. Qualitative aspects." *Early Human Development*, 7(4), 301–322.

De Vries, J. I., Visser, G. H., & Prechtl, H. F. (1985). "The emergence of fetal behaviour. II. Quantitative aspects." *Early Human Development*, 12(2), 99–120.

De Vries, J. I., Visser, G. H., Mulder, E. J., & Prechtl, H. F. (1987). "Diurnal and other variations in fetal movements and heart rate patterns at 20–22 weeks." *Early Human Development*, 15(6), 333–348.

DeCasper, A. J., & Fifer, W. P. (1980). "Of human bonding: newborns prefer their mothers' voices." *Science*, 208(4448), 1174–1176.

DeCasper, A. J., Lecanuet, J.-P., Busnel, M.-C., Granier-Deferre, C., & Maugeais, R. (1994). "Fetal reactions to recurrent maternal speech." *Infant Behavior and Development*, 17(2), 159–164.

DiPietro, J. A., Irizarry, R. A., Costigan, K. A., & Gurewitsch, E. D. (2004). "The psychophysiology of the maternal-fetal relationship." *Psychophysiology*, 41(4), 510–520.

Durier, V., Henry, S., Martin, E., Dollion, N., Hausberger, M., & Sizun, J. (2015). "Unexpected behavioural consequences of preterm newborns' clothing." *Scientific Reports*, 5, 9177.

Fifer, W. P., & Moon, C. M. (1995). "The effects of fetal experience with sound." In: J. P. Lecanuet, W. P. Fifer, N. A. Krasnegor, & W. P. Smotherman (eds.), *Fetal Development: A Psychobiological Perspective*. Hillsdale, NJ: Lawrence Erlbaum Associates. pp. 351–366.

Granier-Deferre, C., Bassereau, S., Ribeiro, A., Jacquet, A.-Y., & DeCasper, A. J. (2011). "A melodic contour repeatedly experienced by human near-term fetuses elicits a profound cardiac reaction one month after birth." *PLoS ONE*, 6(2), e17304.

Henry, M. (2008). *Material Phenomenology*. (S. Davidson, transl.) New York, NY: Fordham University Press. (Original work published 1990).

Henry, M. (2009). *Seeing the Invisible: On Kandinsky*. (S. Davidson, transl.) New York, NY: Continuum. (Original work published 1988).

Hepper, P., Scott, D., & Shahidullah, S. (1993). "Newborn and fetal response to maternal voice." *Journal of Reproductive and Infant Psychology*, 11(3), 147–155.

Hunter, C. J., Bennet, L., Power, G. G., Roelfsema, V., Blood, A. B., Quaedackers, J. S., George, S., Guan, J., & Gunn, A. J. (2003). "Key neuroprotective role for endogenous adenosine A1 receptor activation during asphyxia in the fetal sheep." *Stroke*, 34(9), 2240–2245.

Kawakami, F., & Yanaihara, T. (2012). "Smiles in the fetal period." *Infant Behavior and Development*, 35(3), 466–471.

Kisilevsky, B. S., Hains, S. M., Lee, K., Xie, X., Huang, H., Ye, H. H., Zhang, K., & Wang, Z. (2003). "Effects of experience on fetal voice recognition." *Psychological Science*, 14(3), 220–224.

Lagercrantz, H., & Changeux, J.-P. (2009). "The emergence of human consciousness: from fetal to neonatal life." *Pediatric Research*, 65(3), 255–260.

Latva, R., Lehtonen, L., Salmelin, R. K., & Tamminen, T. (2004). "Visiting less than every day: a marker for later behavioral problems in Finnish preterm infants." *Archives of Pediatrics and Adolescent Medicine*, 158(12), 1153–1157.

Leader, L. R., Baillie, P., Martin, B., & Vermeulen, E. (1982). "The assessment and significance of habituation to a repeated stimulus by the human fetus." *Early Human Development*, 7(3), 211–219.

Lee, G. Y., & Kisilevsky, B. S. (2014). "Fetuses respond to father's voice but prefer mother's voice after birth." *Developmental Psychobiology*, 56(1), 1–11.

Liu, W. F. (2012). "Comparing sound measurements in the single-family room with open-unit design neonatal intensive care unit: the impact of equipment noise." *Journal of Perinatology*, 32(5), 368–373.

Madlinger-Lewis, L., Reynolds, L., Zarem, C., Crapnell, T., Inder, T., & Pineda, R. (2014). "The effects of alternative positioning on preterm infants in the neonatal intensive care unit: a randomized clinical trial." *Research in Developmental Disabilities*, 35 (2), 490–497.

Marlier, L., Schaal, B., & Soussignan, R. (1998). "Neonatal responsiveness to the odor of amniotic and lacteal fluids: a test of perinatal chemosensory continuity." *Child Development*, 69(3), 611–623.

Marx, V., & Nagy, E. (2015). "Fetal behavioural responses to maternal voice and touch." *PLoS ONE*, 10(6), e0129118.

Mellor, D. J., Diesch, T. J., Gunn, A. J., & Bennet, L. (2005). "The importance of 'awareness' for understanding fetal pain." *Brain Research Reviews*, 49(3), 455–471.

Mennella, J. A. (2007). "The chemical senses and the development of flavor preferences in humans." In: T. W. Hale & P. E. Hartmann (eds.), *Hale & Hartmann's Textbook of Human Lactation*. Amarillo, TX: Hale Publishing. pp. 403–414.

Merleau-Ponty, M. (2007). "The child's relations with others." (J. Wild, transl.) In: T. Toadvine & L. Lawlor (eds.), *The Merleau-Ponty Reader*. Evanston, IL: Northwestern University Press. pp. 143–183. (Original work published 1951).

Mirmiran, M., & Ariagno, R. L. (2000). "Influence of light in the NICU on the development of circadian rhythms in preterm infants." *Seminars in Perinatology*, 24(4), 247–257.

Moore, L. M., Persaud, T. V. N., & Torchia, M. G. (2015). *The Developing Human: Clinical Oriented Embryology*. Philadelphia, PA: Saunders.

Ockleford, E. M., Vince, M. A., Layton, C., & Reader, M. R. (1988). "Responses of neonates to parents' and others' voices." *Early Human Development*, 18(1), 27–36.

Pineda, R. G., Neil, J., Dierker, D., Smyser, C. D., Wallendorf, M., Kidokoro, H., Reynolds, L. C., Walker, S., Rogers, C., Mathur, A. M., Van Essen, D. C., & Inder, T. (2014). "Alterations in brain structure and neurodevelopmental outcome in preterm infants hospitalized in different neonatal intensive care environments." *Journal of Pediatrics*, 164(1), 52–60.e2.

Piontelli, A. (2010) *Development of Normal Fetal Movements: The First 25 Weeks of Gestation*. Milan: Springer-Verlag.

Platt, M. W. (2011). "Fetal awareness and fetal pain: the emperor's new clothes." *Archives of Disease in Childhood. Fetal and Neonatal Edition*, 96(4), F236–237.

Potter, E. (1946). "Bilateral renal agenesis." *Journal of Pediatrics*, 29, 68–76.

Querleu, D., Renard, X., Boutteville, C., & Crepin, G. (1989). "Hearing by the human fetus?" *Seminars in Perinatology*, 13(5), 409–420.

Reynolds, L. C., Duncan, M. M., Smith, G. C., Mathur, A., Neil, J., Inder, T., & Pineda, R. G. (2013). "Parental presence and holding in the neonatal intensive care unit and associations with early neurobehavior." *Journal of Perinatology*, 33(8), 636–641.

Sadler, T. W. (2015). *Langman's Medical Embryology*. Philadelphia, PA: Wolters Kluwer Health.

Salk, L. (1973). "The role of the heartbeat in the relation between mother and infant." *Scientific American*, 228(5), 24–29.

Sandman, C. A., Davis, E. P., Buss, C., & Glynn, L. M. (2012). "Exposure to prenatal psychobiological stress exerts programming influences on the mother and her fetus." *Neuroendocrinology*, 95(1), 7–21.

Santos, J., Pearce, S. E., & Stroustrup, A. (2015). "Impact of hospital-based environmental exposures on neurodevelopmental outcomes of preterm infants." *Current Opinion in Pediatrics*, 27(2), 254–260.

Schaal, B., Hummel, T., & Soussignan, R. (2004). "Olfaction in the fetal and premature infant: functional status and clinical implications." *Clinical Perinatology*, 31(2), 261–285.

Schwab, M., Bludau, T., Abrams, R. M., Antonelli, P. J., Gerhard, K. J., & Bauer, R. (1997). "Thermal stimulation of the fetal skin induces ECoG arousal in fetal sheep." *Pflugers Archiv: European Journal of Physiology*, 433(6), 594.

Seidman, G., Unnikrishnan, S., & Kenny, E. (2015). "Barriers and enables of kangaroo mother care practice: a systematic review." *PLoS One*, 10(5), e0125643.

Shahheidari, M., & Homer, C. (2012). "Impact of the design of neonatal intensive care units on neonates, staff, and families: a systemic literature review." *The Journal of Perinatal and Neonatal Nursing*, 26(3), 260–266.

Smith, C. V., Satt, B., Phelan, J. P., & Paul, R. H. (1990). "Intrauterine sound levels: intrapartum assessment with an intrauterine microphone." *American Journal of Perinatology*, 7(4), 312–315.

Smith, J. R. (2012). "Comforting touch in the very preterm hospitalized infant: an integrative review." *Advances in Neonatal Care*, 12(6), 349–365.

Soussignan, R., Schaal, B., Marlier, L., & Jiang, T. (1997). "Facial and autonomic responses to biological and artificial olfactory stimuli in human neonates: re-examining early hedonic discrimination of odors." *Physiology and Behavior*, 62(4), 745–758.

Stevens, D., Thompson, P., Helseth, C., & Pottala, J. (2015). "Mounting evidence favoring single-family room neonatal intensive care." *Journal of Neonatal Perinatal Medicine*, 8 (3), 177–178.

Surenthiran, S. S., Wilbraham, K., May, J., Chant, T., Emmerson, A. J., & Newton, V. E. (2013). "Noise levels within the ear and post-nasal space in neonates in intensive care." *Archives of Disease in Childhood. Fetal and Neonatal Edition*, 88(4), F315–F318.

Valman, H. B., & Pearson, J. F. (1980). "What the fetus feels." *British Medical Journal, 280* (6209), 233–234.

Van Manen, M. A. (2012). "Technics of touch in the neonatal intensive care." *Medical Humanities*, 38(2), 91–96.

Vergara, E. R., & Bigsby, R. (2004). *Developmental and Therapeutic Interventions in the NICU.* Baltimore, MD: Paul H. Brookes Publishing Company.

Voegtline, K. M., Costigan, K. A., Pater, H. A., & DiPietro, J. A. (2013). "Near-term fetal response to maternal spoken voice." *Infant Behavior and Development*, 36(4), 526–533.

Wilkinson, A. R., & Jiang, Z. D. (2006). "Brainstem auditory evoked response in neonatal neurology." *Seminars in Fetal Neonatal Medicine*, 11(6), 444–451.

Yong Ping, E., Laplante, D. P., Elgbeili, G., Hillerer, K. M., Brunet, A., O'Hara, M. W., & King, S. (2015). "Prenatal maternal stress predicts stress reactivity at 2 ½ years of age: the Iowa Flood Study." *Psychoneuroendocrinology*, 56, 62–78.

Zimmer, E. Z., Chao, C. R., Guy, G. P., Marks, F., & Fifer, W. P. (1993). "Vibroacoustic stimulation evokes human fetal micturition." *Obstetrics and Gynecology*, 81(2), 178–180.

3

THE FIRST CRY OF THE CHILD

A baby is born into the world. As the eyes, nose, cheeks, and mouth come into view, the newborn may still appear almost figurine-like in appearance. The face is commonly expressionless, sometimes pinched into a furrowed frown. If the shoulders offer limited resistance, a twist and turn will allow the birthing child to slip out, with a gush of remaining fluid, to lie naked in its entirety. At such a moment, we are confronted with the visibility of the child's body, wet with blood-stained mucous fluid, coated in waxy, white vernix. Still, we have not been 'given' the child.

Slowly and surely arms and legs flex, the baby inhales. The initial short sounds are higher in pitch, sometimes only faintly audible relative to the sounds that follow. Then, the momentous moment happens. In the exhalation is the body and weight of the cry: a full, wet, vibrating holler that calls for more cry. Like the sound of a saw gaining momentum, tone and timbre oscillate irregularly: a coarse spectrum of harmonics. The cry gives the child as self-present. The cry announces the child to the world and to itself.

Humans Cry

Crying is a basic, fundamental, and ubiquitous part of the emotional and behavioral repertoire of human beings (Vingerhoets, 2013). Evolutionary advantageous for the vulnerable newborn, the cry calls for care, support, and protection. Generally, we ascribe crying in the young and adults to negative events: the infant is hungry, the child is not getting his way, the adolescent experiences her relationship ending, or the adult is confronted with the loss of a parent. Sometimes, we may attribute crying to positive events: the infant laughs to the point of crying, the child is overcome with the joy of a gift, the adolescent is caught in the emotion of a first kiss, or the adult is moved to tears when witnessing the amazing accomplishments of a child. Crying is the outward expression on continuums of meaning—anxiety to sentimentality, frustration to pride, and sadness to joy.

Crying, however, is recognized as more than an expression of emotion. Technically, it has been conceptualized as a biopsychosocial phenomenon tempered by biological factors (e.g., physical state, hormonal levels), psychological factors (e.g., demographic and personality factors), and situational social factors (e.g., social norms, location, and presence of others) (Vingerhoets et al., 2000). Developmental psychologists have reported age-related changes in crying across the human lifespan, and linguistic anthropologists have observed cultural differences in crying. But how well do we understand the cry of the young infant and especially the first cry of the newly born? Certainly, there are numerous popular book titles available for new parents that address crying in the young infant: *New Ways to Calm Crying; The Hidden Meaning of Crying; Why is Your Baby Crying? Understanding Your Crying Baby; What Your Crying Child Sees, Feels, and Experiences; Find Out What Your Baby is Thinking.* And yet, although these books often provide advice and recommendations, upon closer examination it becomes quickly clear that the authors take great license with the attribution of meaning to crying. How do we understand the first cry of the newborn child?

The newborn cry is unlike other cries. Its presence does not necessarily signify sorrow or pain for the listening parent. We do not hear regret, worry, or grief— nor is it apparent that the cry expresses the child's pleasure, happiness, or joy. The ones who attend the birth usually respond with a smile to the child's first cry. After all, the baby who takes its first breath must cry, so we think. The first cry is the first sign that a new life has begun. And yet, we should wonder at this cry that the baby seems to perform without having been taught it. The young infant soon learns to imitate many facial and other bodily movements. Indeed, research is increasingly discovering how the young infant is adept at imitation (Lepage & Théoret, 2007). And yet, the first cry is produced without mimesis as the first act of the newborn.

Ancient Romans scripts tell that in the first cry we hear *Vaticanus*, the god who presides over the beginnings of human speech. According to mythology, the cry does not really originate from the child. Rather, the cry is due to *Vaticanus*—the one who opens the mouth of the newborn (*in vagitu*) (Augustine, 2012). The newborn cry is *vitalis*, the cry of life. We hear vitality in the baby's first cry, but what is it that is expressed in this vitality? Or is the first cry not really a matter of expression at all? What else might we hear in the cry? In what sense might the cry be meaningful? How might we constatively reflect on its meaning?

The problem is not that we cannot explain the biological or evolutionary function of the cry; rather, we are puzzled by the enigma of its meaning, both for the child and the adult. Phenomenology leads us back to consider, reflect, and explore the lived meaning of the cry given in its inceptuality, in the primal structures of experience itself. However, can phenomenology adequately address the meaning of the newborn cry—particularly when we recognize that a newborn may experience the world in a vastly different way from the adult, owing to differences in brain, development, and body maturity? Perhaps what we think we hear does not reflect what is experienced? And yet, we do need to consider the newborn's cry.

The Science of the First Cry

Neurobiological studies in animals and humans propose that crying results from a complex interplay of activity of certain brain structures, neurotransmitters, and neurohormones associated with specific psychological states such as helplessness, separation, and pain (Newman, 2007; Parvizi et al., 2009; Pinyerd, 1994). Little, however, is known about the anatomic structures and neurochemical substrates specifically involved in the first cry of the newborn. Instead, the medical literature describes the first cry as physiological: through it, the cardio-respiratory systems transition from fetal to newborn life.

In the womb the fetal lungs are filled with fluid so that in the absence of air no cry may be produced by inhaling-exhaling. Blood is preferentially directed across circulatory shunts, the *foramen ovale* and *ductus arteriosus*, to circumvent the lungs (Rudolph et al., 1988). The *foramen ovale*, the oval opening, allows blood to stream from the right to left filling chambers of the heart; and, the *ductus arteriosus*, the vessel channel, allows blood to flow from the pulmonary artery to the aorta. Since it is the placenta rather than the lungs that provide the means for exchange of oxygen, carbon dioxide, and various other substances, these fetal circulatory shunts ensure that energy is not wasted needlessly, pumping superfluous blood to the lungs.

With the onset and progression of labor, hormone-mediated sodium reabsorption across the pulmonary epithelium and posture-induced increases in transpulmonary pressure contribute to absorption of fetal lung fluid (Hillman et al., 2012). And in a matter of a few seconds to minutes, through a series of interdependent physiological events, the lungs inflate themselves, which prominently contributes to lung fluid absorption (Hooper & Harding, 2005). As the lungs fill with air, the first cry becomes a possibility.

The large inspiration of the cry generates high-pressure, forcing fluid reabsorption (Teitel et al., 1990). Exhalation of the cry is against partially closed vocal cords and related glottic structures, maintaining a progressive establishment of lung inflation (te Pas et al., 2009). Aeration of the lungs in turn triggers a decrease in pulmonary vascular resistance, reversing the pressure gradients across the *foramen ovale* and *ductus arteriosus*, promoting blood flow in the lungs (Crossley et al., 2009; van Vonderen et al., 2014). In crying, blood flow across the ductus into the lungs is further increased in inspiration (van Vonderen et al., 2015). Clamping the umbilical cord at this point severs the umbilical preload volume to the heart and also increases afterload by ceasing the possibility of blood flow from the heart to the low resistance placental circuit (Hooper et al., 2015). We are only now learning that, if clamping does not occur, continued crying can also alter blood flow through the umbilical vein and arteries (Boere et al., 2015). Therefore, it would suggest that it is important to take a physiological approach to the timing of umbilical cord clamping related to such events like crying (Hooper et al., 2015).

From a medical perspective, the first cry expresses vitality, successful transitioning to extra-uterine life, and perhaps even the need to sever the connection of fetus and child. It is not surprising then that the most cardinal of medical assessments for successful fetal transition, the Apgar score, incorporates the first cry whereby the thriving, transitioning infant produces a satisfactory cry: "breathed and cried lustily" (Apgar, 1953, p. 261). The medical first cry has an evolutionary role such that explanation for its occurrence may be reduced to its transitional, and hence survival, benefit. Yet, even while considering the cry as an adaptive, physiological response, we may question what is the sensuality of this adjustment, transition, or change?

The Physiognomy of the First Cry

The sound quality of the cry of the newborn has been studied extensively by acoustic analyses: the spectrographic tracing, the fundamental frequency, the intensity, the duration of emission, the melody, and the presence of different emissions and other sounds. Empirically, the average fundamental frequency of the newborn cry varies around 400 Hz (Fort & Manfredi, 1998; Michelsson & Michelsson, 1999; Wasz-Hökert et al., 1968). The frequency is inversely related to gestational age such that the more immature a newborn is, the higher the pitch of the cry (Goberman & Robb, 1999). When the duration of the cry is considered as the total vocalization that occurs during expiration, it is reported to last from approximately 1 to 1.5 seconds (Robb & Cacace, 1995; Michelsson et al., 2002; Wasz-Hökert et al., 1968). In infants with neurological diseases or congenital syndromes, the frequency of the cry tends to be higher in pitch (Fort & Manfredi, 1998; Michelsson & Michelsson, 1999; Raes et al., 1982). In quick deliveries the cry tends to be strong and acute; in slow deliveries the cry tends to be weak, short, and intermittent (Branco et al., 2005; Makói et al., 1975). Overall it would appear that infants born after vaginal delivery have a longer duration of cry than after caesarean section (Branco et al., 2005).

The first cry does not occur in vocal isolation. Charles Darwin gives a classic description of the crying newborn:

> Whilst thus screaming their eyes are firmly closed, so that the skin round them is wrinkled, and the forehead contracted into a frown. The mouth is widely opened with the lips retracted in a peculiar manner, which causes it to assume a squarish form: the gums or teeth being more or less exposed. The breath is inhaled almost spasmodically.
>
> *(Darwin, 1989, p. 110)*

In the moment of the cry, it is not just the voice that is engaged in the cry. The cry is a full bodily event. The eyes are closed to the world: the newborn does not look to those around him or her. The forehead, brow, and cheeks all contract inwards with the cry: creased, furrowed, and contorted. Down from the face, the trunk flexes, extends, and postures. Arms and legs bend and straighten, in and out of flexion and extension, and even shake. Movements are unrefined, uneven, and crude. There is nothing for the baby to grab or push against. It is not simply that the mouth cries—the body of the newborn cries as limbs move to be settled.

The cry is in stark contrast to a reflex. For example, in the classic newborn 'Moro reflex' the arms symmetrically open and fingers extend in response to a sudden loss of support. For the briefest of moments in the reflex, the body appears caught, fixed, or stuck in a posture of extension, beyond the control of the infant, before he or she is able to bring the arms inward to the chest and close the hands into fists. In comparison, watching a baby cry, we realize that a cry is effortful, expressive, and intentional. Beginning slowly, the inhalation is labored, taken in. Increasing, swelling, or up surging, the inhalation ceases and is briefly held before let out as a cry. The crying may continue with successive determined explosions: each cry escalating in volume and strength to a condition of crying. Considering the effort involved in crying, it is not surprising that the cry has been theorized as a "discharge phenomenon," helping the baby's nervous system regain homeostasis by releasing tension (Brazelton, 1985, p. 332). We can also appreciate how others have interpreted the cry as an attempt to come to terms with one's situation, to strive to achieve emotional balance (Nelson, 2005).

These are the functional theories about the significance of the cry. Functional theories may be significant but they are not necessarily full of meaning. For example, falling in love can be theorized as important for the survival of the species, but that does not mean that humans meaningfully experience or think of species survival in their love life. Similarly, it is clear that the first cry is important for the proper functioning of the organs and blood flow, but it is unclear how this biological-physiological cry is sensually, consciously, or preconsciously engaged by the newborn infant. How infants first cry may be a response to the circumstances of a birthing delivery and how the being of the newborn adapts to the world outside the womb. Based on the above research, it is possible that longer or more complicated deliveries render the baby more exhausted, less able to cry. Alternatively, complications of birth may be physically painful or otherwise unsettling for the newborn and thus intensify the cry. Adaptation (*adaptare*—relating to fitting or adjusting) here is not only a functional-physiological but also a sensual happening (*OED*).

Yet is This the First Cry?

It may be argued that all babies are born premature. More than any other primate species, human babies are dependent on caregivers for life-sustaining care, extending for months to years after birth because capabilities such as vision, hearing, expression, and cognition are immature relative to the adult individual. Thus, we need to be careful to ascribe a special status to the child born at term as being formed complete, whole, in entirety relative to the child born premature. Certainly, premature infants born at the threshold of viability at 23–24 weeks gestation are capable of crying at birth and, while they mature in NICUs, they are observed to engage in newborn behaviors (Giganti et al., 2006). As we question the boundaries between the state of fetus and newborn we may wonder does a fetus cry? And if so, how might such a cry give us constative insights into the meaning of the first cry of the newborn child?

Vagitus uterinus is the name given to the cry that may escape the confines of the uterus (Jackson, 1943; Russell, 1957). In this situation, the soon-to-be-born baby cries before actual birth as a consequence of air entering the uterus and stimulation by tactile manipulation (Kitzmiller & Mitchell, 1942). Such a situation, while being fascinating, is perhaps not at all unexpected because in this situation the cry while happening within the womb actually occurs in the context of a compromised womb: the water has been broken and the soon-to-be-born baby is being touched, stirred, unsettled. But, what about the cry within an intact womb?

Looking within the womb with ultrasound imaging, it is apparent that the fetus has periods of wakefulness, most commonly at night (Patrick et al., 1982; Roberts et al., 1979). These periods of wakefulness, however, consist of active movements that largely seem to be quite unlike any crying behavior observed postnatally with regards to facial expression, movement of the limbs, and measured heart rate (Pillai & James, 1990). It would appear that it is only in the exceptional situation whereby a fetus is provoked that a cry may be incited.

What may be seen by the ultra-sonographer when vibroacoustic stimulation is applied to the mother's abdomen?

There is a brief expiration that is followed by a deep inspiratory phase with a subsequent pronounced expiratory phase. The expiration is associated with jaw opening, taut tongue, and chest depression. It is immediately followed by three augmented breaths with progressively increase in chest rise and head tilt. Each end inspiration is marked by chin quiver. The last augmented breath ends in an inspiratory pause, followed by an expiration and settling. Settling is associated with a turn of the fetal head to the oblique position, mouthing, and swallowing.

(Gingras et al., 2005, pp. F415–F416)

Despite there being a developmental continuity between prenatal and postnatal life, and fetuses having the capacity to cry, crying itself is uncommon for the fetus. The fetal cry is only elicited when the fetus appears disturbed or unsettled (Gingras et al., 2005). So, we are left wondering from such observations whether the newborn first cry is indeed the first cry for a child, and whether the newborn cry is a result of the condition of radical unsettling in being expelled from the womb, that is the birthing event.

The Genesis of the First Cry

In the past, a doctor, midwife, or other attendant to birth would dangle a newborn baby upside down with a firm grip, slapping the rear end to urge a cry. Nowadays, we see a less brusque approach as the baby is actively rubbed down with a towel and the nose and throat are cleared by suction if necessary (Weiner, 2016). Actually, most term babies and even preterm babies cry without any such interventions (O'Donnell et al., 2010). So, phenomenologically we may ask, what gives itself in this first cry and/or how does the first cry give itself to us? Well, the disappointing answer may have to be that the cry does not give itself to us at all. Why? Because the phenomenon of our own birth is inaccessible to us.

> Birth—I am considering here the phenomenon that shows *itself* truly in the mode of what gives *itself*, the properly eventmental phenomenon. In effect, how am I to understand that my birth shows *itself* as a phenomenon, when, properly speaking, I have never seen it with my own eyes and I must rely on eyewitnesses or a birth certificate? Since it is accomplished without me and even, strictly speaking, before me, it should not be able to show *itself* (if it were to show itself) to anyone at all, except to me.
>
> *(Marion, 2002, p. 42, 43)*

One's own birth, considered as a pure event, antedating the first cry, is unavailable to perception except in the pure givenness of its eventuality: "in giving a *me*, a *myself*" (Marion, 2002, p. 43). As adults, we are unable to appreciate birth in its original showing of me to myself. The inceptual existence of the wombed fetus and newborn infant are remote from our memory and possibly even of a qualitatively different, experiential understanding such that the self-givenness and lived meaning of the phenomenal event of our own birth is elusive, inaccessible, or lost.

Many of us may have wondered about the sensuality of birth. Does the birthing event cause or precipitate the first cry? Is there a pain to childbirth not only for the birthing mother but also the child? Does the pressure exerted on the newborn, such as the compressing and distorting of the skull as it descends through the birthing canal, actually cause pain? If such were the case we might expect to see babies routinely inhale to cry and aspirate into the lungs the liquid contents of the vaginal canal. But even when the birth canal is soiled with meconium, it is relatively uncommon that a baby actually develops symptoms to suggest a true meconium aspiration (Fischer et al., 2012; Manganaro et al., 2001).

Buytendijk (1988) has shown that the first smile of the child has a special constative significance that cannot be compared to the smile of the adult.

Paradoxically, in the child's smile is the experience of instability, scintillation, and brightness and yet also the sense of stability, permanence, and closedness. The smile expresses an emerging quality of humanness—the coming into being of the child. Like the first smile, we cannot simply assume that newborns cry for the same reasons as adults. Nor can we assume that our adult words capture what gives rise to the first cry of a child.

The Meaning of the First Cry

Exploring the significance of the first cry tends to orient us to what precedes it and what causes it. But we also need to consider what is subsequent to the cry and what it is that may settle it. Following the first cry, the doctor, midwife, nurse, or other attendant to birth may look to return the child to his or her mother. Returning the child to the mother, placing the child skin-to-skin, seems to calm the first cry. With the arms and legs folded inward, and body held securely, the baby settles and responds to being brought back to a sensuality or holding not unlike the interiority of the womb. But while the first cry is received with joy (that the child is healthily exercising its lungs for the first time), subsequent crying elicits a different response.

Indeed, hearing a baby cry tends to evoke a universal human response. The mother, father, or caregiver cannot ignore the cry, and hearing the cry demands an almost immediate Levinassian gesture: to feel addressed and responsible to care for this vulnerable newborn. Emmanuel Levinas (1969) has shown how the vulnerability of the 'Other' can make a claim on us. The cry of the baby makes us forget our self-preoccupied concerns and calls on us, as parents, to attend to this cry: to check, to touch, to hold the crying newborn. Across diverse cultures, the most common response to infant crying is to pick up the baby, put it to the breast, and/or nurse it (Vingerhoets, 2013). It is as if implicit in the first cry, the first turning of the head and search for the breast, is an intentionality to re-establish comfort, enjoyment, and wellbeing (Simms, 2008). As humans, we seem to be uniquely sensitive to the cry of a crying newborn (Swain et al., 2007).

We recognize existential traces of the texture of the womb world when a newborn calms in response to being held and swaddled, stills in response to the mother's heartbeat, or startles in response to a bright light. During a fetus' inceptual settlement within the womb, the infant has been held in constant contact within a closed interiority of fluid resistance and uterine walls. The repeating and reverberating sounds of heartbeat and other sensual textures composed a wombed life of rhythm for the developing fetus. And of course, the fetus and mother being of a common body create the possibility for fetal perception to be joined to and conditioned by the bodily being of the pregnant mother. The first birthing cry makes possible the subsequent cry, but now not first of all physiological but expressive: expressing a separating or even severing of a womb world existence. Put differently, by way of birth a fetal life turns into a newborn's world that is unsettled. Newly born, the child has been cast into a birthed world—foreign, distant, and external from that which had constituted his or her sense existence as a fetus.

In response to the cry, the mother may whisper soft hushings and other rhythmic sounds or even place the child against her bare chest so that the child is returned to the cadence of the mother's heartbeat and other bodily sounds. With the maternal voice, scents of skin, and taste of breast milk, the newborn may be brought back to a way of fetal being-in-the-world that is closer to the womb. The cry is quieted and soothed. These observations of calming newborn infants' cries are not simply anecdotal but evidenced by clinical research.

It has long been known that almost immediately after birth the newborn, when placed on the mother's chest, displays a rather stereotyped sequence of movements or actions ending at about one hour of age with finding and suckling the nipple (Widström et al., 1987). This behavior is easily disturbed by even minor interventions, resulting in the return or evocation of the first cry. A complementary observation is that when babies are placed in close body contact with their mother after birth, rather than placed in a cot and bundled in blankets, there are virtually no crying episodes in the first 90 minutes postpartum (Christensson et al., 1995). Simple skin-to-skin contact tends to quell the newborn cry (Moore et al., 2016). The first cry is like an "acoustical umbilical cord," maintaining connection between the newborn and mother, abated by the kinaesthetic, tactile, or olfactory stimuli associated with the mother (Ostwald, 1972, p. 352).

The fact that the first cry can be re-aroused through separation or other interruptions of simple or skin-to-skin holding alerts us to a primal, relational meaning that may be the expressivity of the subsequent cry. In such situations, the disturbing or upsetting event that pains could cause an effortful response. Pain not necessarily in the physical sense but rather as an interruption of wombed being and disturbances associated with out-of-womb existence, is new to the newborn and therefore unsettling. We can speculate that the first cry is the expression of an unsettling of the texture of original natality. The cry expresses the loss of womb-child-being—stopping at the reunion of child with mother. The interior settlement of the nurturing womb is traded for the exterior settlement of skin-to-skin existence with the nurturing mother. Still, we may wonder if infants cry not because they are separated from their mother but simply because they have been born from the womb. The first cry of the infant announces the irruption of an interior to an exterior settling, literally occupying a place of settlement into the exterior world.

A Life of Laughing and Crying

In his classic study of *Laughing and Crying*, Plessner (1970) distinguishes several modalities or types of crying. At the elemental level is the crying of the infant that is essentially determined by physiological conditions. The child cries because it is hungry, uncomfortable, painful, alone, and so forth. At the next level is the personal crying that begins in the older child and is characteristic of a deepening of inward experience. For example, the older child may no longer cry when it falls but may cry when the family dog dies. At a more spiritual level there is the weeping that results from deep emotions such as when we are moved to tears by the thing itself, such as a sad story or a poem, and not necessarily with reference to the condition or situation of the personal self. In the mature adult all levels can act up or act together in our conscious existence. Plessner makes subtle distinctions in the way that crying finds its expression in human existence, but he has almost nothing to say about the elemental cry, and even less of the first cry of the newborn child. In fact, he does not even mention the event of the first cry of the newborn.

Of course, it is quite likely that the first cry of the child is 'only' physiological and that it does not yet carry any meaning or significance at all for the child—though it carries highly significant meaning for the caring adult. It is equally likely that the parent who hears the first cry will interpret it as intentional and indicative that the newborn baby is responding negatively to its 'being thrown into the world,' as Heidegger (1962) might say. And soon, when the baby cries the mother or father will immediately presume that the baby is unhappy and needs attention. That is the common response, even if the parent may feel that the baby should not need to cry or should be left to cry for a bit.

Concluding Thoughts

A phenomenological method leads us to question the meaning of the first cry as an expression of unsettling. We do not know whether the newborn actually experiences pain, separation, or distress with the same texture of meaning as a young infant, child, or an adult. Yet we do need to give consideration that the newborn experiences the world differently from the older child or adult not simply because he or she is 'immature,' but rather because birth may indeed give the world to the newborn as an unsettling of its wombed existence.

How should we deal with the crying infant? We recognize that various families and cultures deal with crying very differently. Children who are reared in cultures in which crying is endured or discouraged do not appear to suffer from health or psychological problems at later stages of development—challenging the idea that the reactions to infant crying are decisive for healthy development (Vingerhoets, 2013). Yet if what is expressed in the early cry is an unsettling, are we not always obliged to calm the cry—to hold the newborn so he or she is brought back to the sensuality of womb life?

We may wonder whether as older children or adults, we are ever that distant from our first inceptual cry. The face of the crying adult often seems an expression of infantality: the moistening adult face with tears is reminiscent of the newborn face wet with amniotic fluid; the uncoordinated and almost spasmodic respirations during intense crying may be similar to the initial breathing efforts of the newborn; the closed eyes, wrinkled skin, and open mouth are typical of the crying physiognomy of newborns (Roes, 1989). Should we look on the first cry of the newborn as necessarily different from the crying child or adult? Does the cry of a child or adult not always indicate an unsettling of existence?

References

Apgar, V. (1953). "A proposal for a new method for evaluation of the newborn infant." *Current Researchers in Anesthesia & Analgesia*, 32(4), 260–267.

Augustine. (2012). *The City of God.* (W. Babcock, transl.) Hyde Park, NY: New City Press. (Original work published 426 AD).

Boere, I., Roest, A. A., Wallace, E., Ten Harkel, A. D., Haak, M. C., Morley, C. J., Hooper, S. B., & te Pas, A. B. (2015). "Umbilical blood flow patterns directly after birth before delayed cord clamping." *Archives of Disease in Childhood. Fetal and Neonatal Edition*, 100(2), F121–125.

Branco, A., Behlau, M., & Rehder, M. A. (2005). "The neonatal cry after caesarean section and vaginal delivery during the first minutes of life." *International Journal of Pediatric Otorhinolaryngology*, 69(5), 681–689.

Brazelton, T. B. (1985). "Application of cry research to clinical perspectives." In: B. M. Lester & C. F. Zachariah Boukydis (eds.), *Infant Crying: Theoretical and Research Perspectives*. New York, NY: Plenum Press. pp. 325–340.

Buytendijk, F. J. J. (1988). "The first smile of the child." *Phenomenology + Pedagogy*, 6(1), 15–24.

Christensson, K., Cabrera, T., Christensson, E., Uvnäs-Moberg, K., & Winberg, J. (1995). "Separation distress call in the human neonate in the absence of maternal body contact." *Acta Paediatrica*, 84(5), 468–473.

Crossley, K. J., Allison, B. J., Polglase, G. R., Morley, C. J., Davis, P. G., & Hooper, S. B. (2009). "Dynamic changes in the direction of blood flow through the ductus arteriosus at birth." *The Journal of Physiology*, 587(Pt 19), 4695–4704.

Darwin, C. R. (1989). *The Expression of the Emotions in Man and Animals*. New York, NY: New York University Press. (Original work published 1872).

Fischer, C., Rybakowski, C., Ferdynus, C., Sagot, P., & Gouyon, J. B. (2012). "A population-based study of meconium aspiration syndrome in neonates born between 37 and 43 weeks of gestation." *International Journal of Pediatrics*, 321545.

Fort, A., & Manfredi, C. (1998). "Acoustic analysis of newborn infant cry signals." *Medical Engineering & Physics*, 20(6), 432–442.

Giganti, F., Ficca, G., Cioni, G., & Salzarulo, P. (2006). "Spontaneous awakenings in preterm and term infants assessed throughout 24-h video-recordings." *Early Human Development*, 82(7), 435–440.

Gingras, J. L., Mitchell, E. A., & Grattan, K. E. (2005). "Fetal homologue of infant crying." *Archives of Disease in Childhood. Fetal and Neonatal Edition*, 90(5), F415–418.

Goberman, A. M., & Robb, M. P. (1999). "Acoustic examination of preterm and full-term infant cries: the long-time average spectrum." *Journal of Speech, Language, and Hearing Research*, 42(4), 850–861.

Heidegger, M. (1962). *Being and Time.* (J. Macquarrie, E. Robinson, transl.) New York, NY: Harper & Row. (Original work published 1927).

Hillman, N. H., Kallapur, S. G., & Jobe, A. H. (2012). "Physiology of transition from intrauterine to extrauterine life." *Clinical Perinatology*, 39(4), 769–783.

Hooper, S. B., & Harding, R. (2005). "Role of aeration in the physiological adaptation of the lung to air breathing at birth." *Current Respiratory Medicine Reviews*, 1(2), 185–195.

Hooper, S. B., Polglase, G. R., & te Pas, A. B. (2015). "A physiological approach to the timing of umbilical cord clamping at birth." *Archives of Disease in Childhood. Fetal and Neonatal Edition*, 100(4), F355–360.

Jackson, I. M. (1943). "Cry of the child in utero." *British Medical Journal*, 2(4312), 266–267.

Kitzmiller, J. L., & Mitchell, W. B. (1942). "Vagitus uterinus." *Western Journal of Surgery, Obstetrics, and Gynecology*, 50, 620–621.

Lepage, J. F., & Théoret, H. (2007). "The mirror neuron system: grasping others' actions from birth?" *Developmental Science*, 10(5), 513–523.

Levinas, E. (1969). *Totality and Infinity: An Essay on Exteriority*. (A. Lingis, transl.) Pittsburgh, PA: Duquesne University Press. (Original work published 1961).

Makói, Z., Szöke, Z., Sasvári, L., Kiss, G., & Popper, P. (1975). "The first cry of the newborn following vaginal delivery or cesarean section." *Acta Paediatrica Academiae Scientiarum Hungaricae*, 16(2), 155–161.

Manganaro, R., Mamì, C., Palmara, A., Paolata, A., & Gemelli, M. (2001). "Incidence of meconium aspiration syndrome in term meconium-stained babies managed at birth with selective tracheal intubation." *Journal of Perinatal Medicine*, 29(6), 465–468.

Marion, J-L. (2002). *In Excess: Studies of Saturated Phenomenon*. (R. Horner, V. Berrand, transl.) New York, NY: Fordham University Press. (Original work published 2001).

Michelsson, K., & Michelsson, O. (1999). "Phonation in the newborn, infant cry." *International Journal of Pediatric Otorhinolaryngology*, 49(Supp 1), S297–S301.

Michelsson, K., Eklund, K., Leppänen, P., & Lyytinen, H. (2002). "Cry characteristics of 172 healthy 1- to 7-day-old infants." *Folia Phoniatrica et Logopaedica*, 54(4), 190–200.

Moore, E. R., Bergman, N., Anderson, G. C., & Medley, N. (2016). "Early skin-to-skin contact for mothers and their healthy newborn infants." *Cochrane Database of Systematic Reviews*, 11, CD003519.

Nelson, J. K. (2005). *Seeing Through Tears: Crying and Attachment*. New York, NY: Brunner-Routledge.

Newman, J. D. (2007). "Neural circuits underling crying and cry responding in mammals." *Behavioural Brain Research*, 182(2), 155–165.

O'Donnell, C. P., Kamlin, C. O., Davis, P. G., & Morley, C. J. (2010). "Crying and breathing by extremely preterm infants immediately after birth." *Journal of Pediatrics*, 156 (5), 846–847.

Ostwald, P. (1972). "The sounds of infancy." *Developmental Medicine & Child Neurology*, 14 (3), 350–361.

Parvizi, J., Coburn, K. L., Shillcutt, S. D., Coffey, C. E., Lauterbach, E. C., & Mendez, M. F. (2009). "Neuroanatomy of pathological laughing and crying: a report of the American Neuropsychiatric Association Committee on Research." *Journal of Neuropsychiatry and Clinical Neurosciences*, 21(1), 75–87.

Patrick, J., Campbell, K., Carmichael, L., Natale, R., & Richardson, B. (1982). "Patterns of gross foetal body movements over 24-hour observation intervals during the last 10 weeks of pregnancy." *Obstetrics & Gynecology*, 142(4), 363–371.

Pillai, M., & James, D. (1990). "Are the behavioural states of the newborn comparable to those of the foetus?" *Early Human Development*, 22(1), 39–49.

Pinyerd, B. J. (1994). "Infant cries: physiology and assessment." *Neonatal Network*, 13(4), 15–20.

Plessner, H. (1970). *Laughing and Crying: A Study of the Limits of Human Behaviour*. Evanston, IL: Northwestern University Press.

Raes, J., Michelsson, K., Dehaen, F., & Despontin, M. (1982). "Cry analysis in infants with infectious and congenital disorders of the larynx." *International Journal of Pediatric Otorhinolaryngology*, 4(2), 157–169.

Robb, M. P., & Cacace, A. T. (1995). "Estimation of formant frequencies in infant cry." *International Journal of Pediatric Otorhinolaryngology*, 32(1), 57–67.

Roberts, A. B., Little, D., Cooper, D., & Campbell, S. (1979). "Normal patterns of fetal activity in the third trimester." *British Journal of Obstetrics and Gynaecology*, 86(1), 4–9.

Roes, F. L. (1989). "On the origin of crying and tears." *Human Ethology Newsletter*, 5(10), 5–6.

Rudolph, A. M., Iwamoto, H. S., & Teitel, D. F. (1988). "Circulatory changes at birth." *Journal of Perinatal Medicine*, 16(suppl 1), 9–21.

Russell, P. M. (1957). "Vagitus uterinus; crying in utero." *Lancet*, 272(6960), 137–138.

Simms, E. (2008). *The Child in the World: Embodiment, Time, and Language in Early Childhood*. Detroit, MI: Wayne State University Press.

Swain, J. E., Lorberbaum, J. P., Kose, S., & Strathearn, L. (2007). "Brain basis of early parent–infant interactions: psychology, physiology, and in vivo functional neuroimaging studies." *Journal of Child Psychology and Psychiatry*, 48(3–4), 262–287.

Te Pas, A. B., Wong, C., Kamlin, C. O., Dawson, J. A., Morley, C. J., & Davis, P. G. (2009). "Breathing patterns in preterm and term infants immediately after birth." *Pediatric Research*, 65(3), 352–356.

Teitel, D. F., Iwamoto, H. S., & Rudolph, A. M. (1990). "Changes in the pulmonary circulation during birth-related events." *Pediatric Research*, 27(4 Pt 1), 372–378.

Van Vonderen, J. J., Roest, A. A., Walther, F. J., Blom, N. A., van Lith, J. M., Hooper, S. B., & te Pas, A. B. (2015). "The influence of crying on the ductus arteriosus shunt and left ventricular output at birth." *Neonatology*, 107(2), 108–112.

Van Vonderen, J. J., te Pas, A. B., Kolster-Bijdevaate, C., van Lith, J. M., Blom, N. A., Hooper, S. B., & Roest, A. A. (2014). "Non-invasive measurements of ductus arteriosus flow directly after birth." *Archives of Disease in Childhood. Fetal and Neonatal Edition*, 99 (5), F408–F412.

Vingerhoets, A. D. (2013). *Why Only Humans Weep: Unravelling the Mysteries of Tears*. Oxford: Oxford University Press.

Vingerhoets, A. J. J. M., Cornelius, R. R., van Heck, G. L., & Becht, M. C. (2000). "Adult crying: a model and review of the literature." *Review of General Psychology*, 4(4), 354–377.

Wasz-Hökert, O., Lind, J., Partanem, T., Vallane, E., & Vuorenkoski, V. (1968). "The infant cry: a spectrographic and auditory analysis." *Clinics in Developmental Medicine*, 29, 1–42.

Weiner, G. M. (ed.). (2016). *Textbook of Neonatal Resuscitation, 7th Edition*. Elk Grove Village, IL: American Academy of Pediatrics.

Widström, A.-M., Ransjö-Arvidson, A.-B., Christensson, K., Matthiesen, A.-S., Winberg, J., & Uvnäs-Moberg, K. (1987). "Gastric suction in the newborn infants: effects on circulation and developing feeding behaviours." *Acta Paediatrica Scandinavica*, 76, 566–572.

4

THE MEANING OF EXTREMELY PREMATURE INFANT BEHAVIOR

Caring for children who are born extremely premature requires close attendance in way clinical examination and during other kinds of interventions. After all, healthcare professionals need to assess and monitor the wellbeing of these fragile infants for possible clinical complications of prematurity and the needed medical treatments used to manage them.

As the physician examines Jon, he opens his eyes, casting darted looks. His body moves in sharp, wriggling twists. With each palpation of his abdomen he turns more flushed, arching his back. His breathing pauses momentarily only to quicken and then pause again. And as the exam continues, his face darkens in redness. His body and limbs turn limp. Breathing pauses, and his eyes close. Redness becomes cyanosis as heart rate and saturations fall.

While examination may be focused on better understanding the integrity or disease of a particular organ system such as the lungs, heart, intestines, and so forth, neurobehavioral assessment is regarded as a needed holistic approach to understand the wellbeing of infants (Lean et al., 2017). One example is Newborn Individualized Developmental Care and Assessment Program. The theoretical basis of this program is based upon the Synactive Theory of Development whereby the behavioral organization of premature infants is described in terms of autonomic, motor, and state subsystems that are in a constant condition of inter-action (Als, 1982). The development and relations of these systems are considered immature such that too much (or too little) stimulation can unsettle the physiologic stability and behavioral organization of the newborn. From this theoretical perspective, premature infants are conceptualized to have an "organizational agenda" (Als & Brazelton, 1981, p. 242). It is only over time that infants develop the ability to regulate themselves to effectively hold themselves together in response to their environment (Als, 1977).

The premature infant's environment has to be understood in a broad manner. Everything structures and impacts on the infant, including the presence of caregivers, the supporting technologies, the background infrastructure, and so forth. Both the quality and quantity of interactions are significant. This ecological perspective of behavior organization guides clinicians, researchers, and parents in their understanding of the ways newborns mature: the coordination of breathing, sucking, and swallowing; the capacity to move food down into and through the gastrointestinal tracks without upwards reflux or vomiting; the ability to interact with caregivers while maintaining regulation in body tone; as well as other developmental accomplishments. However, the neonatal synactive discipline of using primarily behavioral observations and focusing on external appearances may be less attentive to possible affective and meaning dimensions of infant behaviors. Focusing on the behaviors and the physiology of the corporeal body may discourage looking at the body as the center of sensory experience and sensuality. Many years ago, the French philosopher Maurice Merleau-Ponty (1963) warned that behavioral observation may act as a perceptual blinker: when a scientific psychological methodological perspective restricts interpretations of observations to cognitive or behavioristic paradigms, it is possible that the character and meaning of such behaviors are not seen (p. 219).

Emotional reactions and sensations not only result from situation-determined effects, they also well up from primal bodiliness such as fatigue, hunger, pain, and so forth (Buytendijk, 1974). We recognize such effects in the overly tired child who cannot help but suffer a melt-down, or the child who becomes more agreeable after having a snack. Physiologic changes have consequences for emotional-life, which are expressive of a meaningful bodily being-in-the-world. From a phenomenological physiologic perspective, we need to *read* autonomic, motor, and state changes as animating and also expressing the experiential meanings that inhere in behavior.

As previously mentioned, the challenge for studying the lived experience of the premature infant is that in trying to intuit the subjectivity of an infant, our own adult subjectivity inevitably seems to serve as the main source of inspiration. Even the everyday language of caregivers reflects such a tendency. In response to a crying child, we readily attribute the behavior as if it were expressing unified sensations ('Your bum feels dirty?'), first personal authorship ('You want the soother?'), and/or motives-goals ('You are crying so mommy will not leave?'). As Stern (1985) writes:

> Parents thus view young infants on the one hand as physiological systems in need of regulation and, on the other hand, as fairly developed people with subjective experiences, social sensibilities, and a sense of self that is growing, if not already in place.

(p. 43)

However, the subjectivity of the newborn should not be taken as simply premature, growing in equivalence to that of the adult. Instead, we need to recognize that the meaning the world has for an infant, at any given point in time, depends not simply on emergent perceptual and motor capacities, but also on the learning that has already happened and that is occurring now (Johnson, 2007). Developmental psychology tends to skirt this issue by asking, 'What *can* an infant see, hear, smell, or touch?' But such evasion leaves lacunae in our understandings of how to respond to the question, 'What *does* an infant see, hear, smell, or touch?' When addressing the subjectivity of the premature infant, we need to start from an understanding of perception. Rather than regarding behaviors of prematurely born infants as 'disordered' and 'disorganized' we need to qualify these terms as soon as we employ them. Disordered and disorganized behavior is the perception of the healthcare professional who sees no order in the infant's movements and behavior. We should ask, how is disorder organized in the (professional's) perception that only sees disorder? In what way is the disorder ordered in the perception or the object of the (dis)ordered perception? In going beyond the conceptual boundary of Synactive Theory, we ask, what orders the disorder in the behavior of infants born premature? We might ask, what is the possible meaningful (dis)order of the behavior we observe? But the point is that we observe already more than mere behavior. As a starting point for constative reflection, let us attend to close observations of infants born extremely premature at less than 28 weeks gestation, and cared for within the NICU.

Lacking Contact

When the nurse checks on Rose, she finds her active with legs kicking unevenly. The heart rate is 174, rather high. Rose shakes her head vigorously, with sporadic pauses. She momentarily mouths at the bedding or simply makes mouthing movements in the air. Nothing else appears to be within grasp. Aware of the fuss, the nurse opens the isolette and administers a soother. Rose spits it out. The nurse adds a few drips of milk before trying again. This time Rose takes the soother more readily. While this is happening, the nurse places her hand to brace and hold Rose's feet. Her body seems to relax. Eyes close as she drifts into a slumber.

Like Rose, we encounter the world in a feeling way. Our bodies literally come up against surfaces, contours, margins, edges, and all manner of planes by way of our fingers, lips, hands, arms, legs, and trunk. Whether we lie prone, crouch, sit, stand, walk, or run we are always in feeling contact with the world. And, of course, we also feel the world through our eyes, ears, and mouths. Merleau-Ponty (1968) calls this our "perceptual world," emphasizing that our perspective of the world is anchored in our bodily being-in-the-world (p. 170).

Now, consider the premature infant, whose body shudders and flails. As legs and arms move through motions of extension, the outward observational appearance is of limbs failing to meet that for which they feel—a surface, a boundary, or a limit. The open mouth similarly appears to lack, calming not simply with touch but rather with a particular sense of taste. Is 'disorganization' truly the correct word to describe such movements? First, should we not consider the so-called disordered and disorganized behavior of the infant actually perfectly ordered and organized? The constatation is that the infant who fusses and grimaces is expressing in a naturally ordered manner a condition of which we need to be aware. Second, should we not wonder whether these so-called disordered and disorganized movements have a meaningful or an intentional quality to them?

> Daniel lies awake and fusses, tucked into flexion by a white rolled-up sheet, covered with a light cloth. His back arches repeatedly, head and arms shake, and his right foot pushes against the roll. Although his face is contorted in cry, no sound is heard. Mechanically ventilated, the breathing tube impedes his voice. Between periods of crying and fussing, his body turns still as he breathes irregularly fast, skin sucking in between his ribs. When his mother speaks to him, holding his hand, Daniel briefly becomes less squirmy, before again arching, twisting his body, raising his arms into the air, and spreading out his fingers. His face reddens as he extends his right foot, pushing against the roll. His nurse pulls the roll in more tightly around him before putting her hands firmly onto his body. For several minutes, Daniel stops moving, turns less red in the face. As he drifts into sleep, he makes a few sucking movements on his breathing tube.

From a bodily being-in-the-world, we feel the world such that not only do we grasp the world, but the world also grasps us in contact. We find ourselves touched in a particular way that reflects not only the original intent of our touch but also the manner in which we experience the touching, suggests Merleau-Ponty (1962). For example, for the young child or adult, the experience of walking is at once both the experience of striking the ground and also feeling the ground in the strike of the feet. Such contact, a feeling of the resistance of the world, is given immediately in a non-reflective way—meaning, we tend not to think of the experience of walking so much as we just walk about, carrying out our day-to-day activities. Similarly, once comfortable or settled in a chair, our awareness of the texture, firmness, and cushion constitutes nothing more than background awareness to our being in the chair. Yet, deliberate or not, we occasionally shift our position in response to possible pressure points of constant contact. Such shifts in position are not simply due to feelings of sweatiness, heat, achiness, discomfort, or otherwise feelings of disturbance in our being; but also feelings of absence or a lack as we press against a cushion or the ground to sense the firmness of resistance.

But feeling the physicality of the world may come up unexpectedly empty if a chair were to give way. While walking, we may fail to anticipate unevenness in the pavement or walkway. We miss a step, and perhaps trip, stumble, or fall. And in that ephemeral moment before striking the pavement we experience the 'step in its absence' as our body shudders and flails. For the briefest stretch of experience, we are without contact, our body is not touching anything. Contact means touch, in touchness. Yet to be without touch is not simply a lack of physical sensation as we feel when we jump into the air without touching anything. It is true that, in the jump, there is not a feeling of contact until our feet hit the ground. But, in the moment of jumping, falling, or stumbling, the 'step in its absence' refers to the chiasmic nature of the experience. The chiasmic movement is in itself incomplete because it lacks kinship between the sentient and the sensible (Merleau-Ponty, 1968). There is merely a failed feeling for touch, a lacking of contact.

Premature infants, of course, neither walk nor sit in chairs. Still, they do come from a place of constant contact—the inceptual beginning of being enwombed within the womb. However, the infants in the NICU have left the wombed existence such that we may assume that traces of the sensuality of the womb are only brought back to presence when the child is held in containment, when maternal tastes meet the lips, when rhythmic sounds are feelingly heard, and so forth. Without such constant contact, the shuddering and flailing body can only grasp at air as intentionality fails to sense its object, coming up empty in search of its directedness. It is thus not surprising that it has long been observed that premature infants extend, flex, shake, and so forth most in the days initially following birth (Nilsson, 1973). They are literally falling: failing to feel the primal resistance of the physicalness of the womb, denied inceptual touch of the primal cradle of existence.

Emma utters frequent whimpering sounds. Every couple of minutes, she squirms, moves her body and turns quite red in the face. She arches her back and then sighs before settling back into what appears as a restless sleep.

Emma seems to lack something. But what sense of lack could mark such moments? How disturbing is lacking wombed contact for a premature infant? The question is not so much, does a premature infant experience anxiety, nervousness, or insecurity? But rather, can we recognize the possibility that, what theory calls 'disordered behavior' is movement that expresses an active feeling for contact that constantly comes up unfulfilled, deficient, or lacking? In other words, the constatational insight is that this seeming disorder actually has order. Phenomenologically, this is the uneasy moment of a fall, stumble, or other experience where contact is lacking, sensing that it is not just contact with *objects* but also with *subjects* that can be lacking. And if we can imagine the possibility for such experiential meaning, what is the significance of not just one shuddering movement but rather shudder after shudder after shudder after shudder? It may be that the infant not only experiences a restless sleep such that he or she will awaken weary, spent, and tired; but also, the living experience of being is without resting in, on, or against something that would give the infant in-touchness.

Unsettling Stimulation

> Closing her eyes will not shut out the light on her face. And with each pass of the light, her skin color turns more and more dusky, her breathing turns faster and more irregular. When light is flashed in front of her, she shows a second phase to her response such that after several seconds, she squirms, twitches her hands, and then stops breathing for a few seconds before going back to her baseline. By the end of the series of light flashes, her mouth has fallen open. Her hands remain where they had been—clenched just in front of her mouth.

What meaning does sensuality have for infants in these moments of so-called 'disordered behavior'? Cognitive-behaviorists might use words such as 'stimuli' to describe the instants of light, sound, or touch that incite, trigger, or cause a response. And while the term 'stimulus' names that what stimulates, the value of its objectivity passes over the subjective meaning that inheres in any flash, point, prick, or other sensory provocation.

Experiences are not necessarily simple, defined events for infants, involving each of the primary senses. They likely consist of (amodal or multimodal) textures that transcend any single sensory modality (Johnson, 2007; Stern, 1985). For example, for the newborn the voice that whispers in repetition "Shhhh, Shhhh, Shhhh" may be experientially fused with the hand that touches "Pat, Pat, Pat." While we cannot ask an infant what it is like to be disturbed from sleep, it is a recognizable experience for any young child or adult lying in bed or drearily awakening. In response to morning light or noise, the sleeping person may be inclined to roll over, cover the eyes with a blanket, or simply let out a protesting expression. For the sleeper the world is reduced to the bed: "to the spot where his body lies, perhaps even to that little spot where his head rests on the pillow and where he finds space to breathe" (van den Berg, 1966, p. 62). External stimulation is not simply sensed as light, sound, or touch; but rather, as an interruption, break, or disturbance of being. The stimulation is disruptive of sleep; otherwise, it truly would not be stimulating.

While a young child or adult may be able to shut such stimuli out, a premature infant is usually unable to limit the exposure to the flux of disrupting sensuality, let alone willfully control his or her response to the world—the body seemingly cannot help but respond.

> The noise of a rattle leads to the same pattern of color change, increased breathing rate usually follows after some seconds, by a squirmy movement of her body, with occasional grunting and bearing down, going red, then a pause in her breathing. With the final rattle, she gags and her heart rate drops causing her monitor to alarm.

Stimulation is meaningful in its meaninglessness. Its phenomenality as stimulation does not sink into our background awareness as we would expect with what we have habituated to. Instead, stimulation is significant in its spur. Yet, it is also meaningless in that it does not follow from an anticipated event. Pain is perhaps the most classic of stimuli because no matter what we tell ourselves, watch in anticipation, or otherwise prepare ourselves for a painful prick, it is always given as a disrupting sensation associated at the very least with a sting. So, we may constatively wonder how the theoretical concept 'disordered behavior' is expressive not simply of external stimulation but more significantly of an intrusive disruption, or disturbance, such that the premature infant exists in a state of constant need for recovery.

> After another few minutes of holding her snugly swaddled with her hands near her mouth and giving her my finger to hold, I jiggle a small toy that produces some soft "tinkles." Emma responds after a few "tinkles" of the toy, by changing her expression in a similar way but she does not open her eyes. By this time, her breathing pattern is more irregular with longer pauses. These pauses are not long enough to trigger her monitor alarm but they are more frequent than those seen in the beginning of the exam. The color around her eyes and mouth is more grey. It seems that Emma is tired and needs a break.

The premature infant, unable to tolerate stimulation, relies on the adult to give him or her a rest. Such a constative insight is important because we need to recognize that disordered behavior expresses an unsettling that a premature infant may be unable to recover from without the support of a caregiver. More profoundly perhaps we need to consider that what is expressed in disordered behavior is, in some respect, not unlike pain.

To be sure, we need to be careful not to hazard that the premature infant needs an environment that lacks stimulation. But one does need to consider how infants may only be able to focus briefly, apparently needing to take a short break by looking or turning away, closing their eyes, yawning, becoming mildly drowsy. The presence of stimulation demands energy and effort, and perhaps may be facilitated if it can be introduced within an experiential structure of expectant primal experiences. Premature infants are not static in their development. They exist in a world that is "becoming meaningful to them" (Johnson, 2007, p. 33).

Exposed Bodiliness

> She starts to bend her neck backwards, and pushes out her right arm, almost pushing herself up off the bed with that arm. She then tucks herself forward, turning more red and grey around the mouth. The fingers of her right hand open up and repeatedly clench into a fist while making these movements. Her heart rate shoots up to 202, setting off the monitor alarm, bringing her nurse to her bedside to silence it. Next her heart rate drops back down to about 170 and then her blood

oxygen levels drops briefly to 79, before returning to the high 90's. She is not moving her body now, her heart rate drops further to 91, and the oxygen level again to 79, setting off the monitor alarms again and bringing her nurse back to her bedside. Her skin is mottled, and her mouth hangs completely open.

In the NICU, it is not unusual to see a premature infant in a reprise of instability in bodily tone, breathing, and circulation. While it is possible such 'disorder' relates 'simply' to prematurity, it is also possible that a compromising medical condition is evolving. We know that the presentation of instability may be seen in older infants who possess 'limited reserve.' For these medically fragile infants the use of medications for sedation may be necessary to keep them calm, for fear of their incapacity to tolerate physiologic lability. One wonders: how do infants experience bodily fluctuations?

Emotions arise from and give rise to bodily states (Lang, 1994). For example, our body reacts to a sudden startle with muscle tightening, quickened breath, and increased heart rate. But the arousal from a startle usually does not immediately dissipate subsequent to the event. Instead, we stay awakened, roused, or even on edge. When a premature infant experiences sudden fluctuations in tone, breathing, and circulation, we need to wonder how do these ecological-physiologic variations affect the lived through experience of such events. The concern is not simply limited to an infant's bodiliness but also bodiliness as it is shared with others.

Rosy is lifted out of the incubator and gently placed against her mother's bare chest. Rosy squirms, flaying her arms and legs. As the monitoring wires and intravenous lines are neatly being gathered by her nurse, the mother leans back a bit more as she places her left hand over Rosy's head. Now Rosy flexes her body, bringing a hand to her mouth. Her heart rate and breathing become steady.

The boundary between body and environment cannot be sharply drawn (Merleau-Ponty, 1968). We are open onto the world, embedded within it and of it, such that sound, light, heat, taste, and touch constitute our very bodily being. For example, the blind person feels the sidewalk through the cane, the dentist appreciates the hardness of enamel through the probe, and the astronomer sees distant stars as near through the telescope—with all of these embodied technologies the world is given anew as part of the body (Ihde, 1990).

It is unclear to what extent a premature infant experiences objects or others in their distinctness within their environment. For example, given a newborn's capacity for amodal or multimodal perception, the breast may be encountered as part of the sensuality of familiarity, possibly without being constituted as a purely visual, tactile, or chemostatic entity. While the taste of breast milk may arouse a familiarity, it is unclear if or how a newborn appreciates how different is the texture of familiarity provided by the taste of breast milk in comparison with the familiarity provided by the mother's voice. In other words, how does the new-born make sense of breast and mother, and are these sensualities experienced in a fused manner or given distinctively?

Stern has posited that the subjective experience of the newborn encompasses an "emergent sense of self" (Stern, 1985, p. 45). If this is true then the infant's world is formed by separate experiences that may lack relatedness. But when diverse experiences are being associated, assimilated, or connected, the infant may experience the emergence of organization. The question is whether the infant may subsequently also experience disorganization? In other words, are organization and disorganization dependent on each other?

> Jacob's mother arrives. She looks preoccupied and worried. "I only have a couple of hours and should do kangaroo care. I know it's important." As the nurse and respiratory therapist move Jacob to her, it is apparent that mother is trying to relax, yet neither Jacob nor his mother settle down, both are constantly shifting position.

Neonatology increasingly recognizes the benefits of skin-to-skin care for infants and their caregivers. Although there is no doubt that holding and close contact are overall good for premature infants, we also need to recognize that infants can become infected with stress when held by someone who is restless or tense. It is evident from studies of older infants and their parents that an infant's physiological state may be influenced by their parent's condition of stress (Waters et al., 2014). The point is that infants are physiologically and emotionally open to the world. And perhaps more importantly, premature infants are even more at the mercy of the parent's physiology that may impact the infant body. In other words, if there is disorder to an infant's behavior, we need to understand where and how the order of such disorder may actually originate.

Regaining Equanimity

> As they slowly remove the tapes securing the breathing tube to his cheeks, Daniel wakes, He arches his back and shakes his head from side-to-side. His face is reddened. As the breathing tube is withdrawn, Daniel appears to struggle to breathe. Bubbled secretions are suctioned as his heart rate slows and oxygen levels drop. As an oxygen mask is snugly held, Daniel takes only occasional gasping breaths. The respiratory therapist gives breaths by mask and now heart rate and blood oxygen respond. Daniel begins to breathe although still slow and irregular. A CPAP mask is fitted before Daniel is gently rolled onto his tummy. His body is limp, his face is dusky-grey, and his mouth is drooped open. Daniel's father puts his hand on Daniel's legs, cupping his fingers around Daniel's feet. Mother crosses her wrists placing her hands firmly over his body. Daniel's breathing is gurgled and raspy but it slowly settles. Over the next few minutes, Daniel starts to open and close his

eyes. His breathing becomes a little less labored and the dark grey tones of his face become less obvious.

A caregiver who attempts to settle a fussing infant may offer a soother. Or some feed may be given. Or quite simply, the child may be held—arms and legs tucked in, gently rocking and a whispering voice. Such attentive gestures of caregivers are common responses to the restless premature infant.

Beneath the blanket, Sara squirms in her sleep—arching her back, stretching out her arms, and fanning her fingers. Sara's mother gently uncovers her blanket, holds her hand and strokes her back. As the legs of the sleeper are uncovered, Sara yawns. Her body produces a few twitches and she stretches backward and extends her arms and legs repeatedly. Her mother talks softly as she checks the diaper, wipes her bottom, and applies some cream. During this time, Sara gradually gains a quiet alertness. Her mother puts on a new diaper. As she leaves Sara's bedside to throw the old diaper away and sanitize her hands, Sara kicks her legs then stretches out her legs straight up into the air. Sara attempts to bring her hand to her mouth. She becomes fussy, produces some sounds, and then her legs limply fall onto the bed. When mother returns she wraps Sara in a blanket and picks her up. She offers her a bottle and Sara starts to suck. Sara gazes at her mother's face, as she is softly spoken to.

We need to ask what is gained or potentially lost when we label a child's behavior as disordered. It is clearly important not to confuse such behaviors with seizures or other medical pathology. Also, it is important to recognize the developmental trajectory of premature infants—they need particular supports for their development. The caregiving developmental question is, where is a premature infant in his or her developmental trajectory, and what should we be doing to support further development? From a basic human perspective of understanding, however, we also constantly need to reflect on and be attentive to the nature and possibilities of meaningful experiences: what may this child's life be like right here and now? "We simply do not know if infants are actually feeling what their faces, voices, and bodies so powerfully express to us, but it is very hard to witness such expressions and not to make that inference," says Stern (1985, p. 66).

Ordered Disorder and Organized Disorganization

Reflecting on the above observational accounts of so-called disordered and disorganized behaviors of infants born extremely premature poses a special challenge for neonatology. How should we interpret and understand such observations? And what sense can we make of these behaviors that in the neonatal literature are termed 'disorganized' and 'disordered'? Observations of the behaviors of premature infants are so primal that it would be a mistake to interpret them in the same way as we might do with observations of infants born more mature. Calling the behaviors of premature infants 'disordered' and 'disorganized' may be an attempt to stay objective and refuse to speculate or interpret meanings. And yet, we should realize that calling such behaviors 'disordered' and 'disorganized' is already an interpretation, namely to refuse to admit that there might be order and organization and that these might be meaningful.

Whether we like it or not, we tend to read behavioral accounts of premature babies empathically. But, we need to be careful that we do not submit to inter-subjective sensitivities that are rooted in faulty empathic presumptions. We need to question our own adult perspective. Should the question be: what is it that the infants' faces, voices, and bodies seem to express? Reading the behavioral accounts of premature infant behaviors is evocative at a pathic embodied level—where pathic understandings are gained intuitively. The term 'pathic' implicates forms of expressive understanding that are rooted in empathy and sympathy and that involve imaginatively placing oneself in someone else's shoes, feeling what the other person feels, understanding the other from a distance or, more generally, to be understandingly engaged in other people's lives. But these relational linguistic notions also open up ways of thinking about expressivity and forms of understanding that are more direct and intuitive. No doubt, there are various forms and modalities of pathic understanding. But the first important point is that the terms empathy and sympathy suggest that this understanding is not primarily theoretic, cognitive, intellectual, technical—but rather that it is indeed pathic: involving the emotions, the body, and pathic sensitivity.

When perceiving an infant kicking and flailing its limbs we perceive or grasp an intentionality of that newborn's world. In other words, we do not identify this kicking the feet into the air with our own behavior because we do not do that as adults. We do not project our own experiential sense of kicking and flailing our limbs since that is not our adult experience. Rather than seeing these behaviors as expressive and inferring certain causes or motives, we need to gain an empathic understanding that is more direct and immediate, before we even ask inferential questions. So, we do not need to assign certain emotions such as sadness or anger to the behaviors but nonetheless may 'understand' the rich sensuality or sensual contents of the physical movement of the flailing arms, the kicking feet, the clenching hands, the sucking mouths that are already meaningful in their felt intentionality. It is the infant's way of being prematurely in the world that is beset with the order of premature intentionalities. The task then for the clinician, researcher, or parent is to attend to the possible affective and meaning aspects of newborn behaviors rather than reduce such meaning to abstract cognitive or behavioristic paradigms.

Concluding Thoughts

Observing the behaviors of infants who are born extremely premature and theorizing about the organized degree of disorganization of these behaviors prematurely commits us to a perspective that ironically compromises a sensitive understanding of prematurity. Yet speculation on the significance of behavior mirrors back to us what we already infer. Phenomenologists such as Husserl (1989), Stein (1989), and Zahavi (2014), have pointed out that inferential observations and projection of one's own experiences onto others' behaviors are based on faulty premises. Inferring a feeling or emotion based on an observed expression and projecting onto the other person (the baby) the meaning of a feeling based on our own emotions leaves us trapped in our own adult experience and world. Understanding the inner life of premature infants does not require that we presume the same emotions that we possess ourselves. We do not know intellectually or speculatively whether, how, or what it is that infants are actually experiencing. Yet, if we observe these behaviors pathically and not just externally then we may tentatively grasp their inceptual meanings. Indeed, if we do not pathically wonder about the experiential life of the newborn we may jeopardize care that is founded in compassion and understanding.

The next chapter moves on to explore the nature of our intersubjective relation with newborns by asking if indeed the newborn actually can see?. Can the newborn already see meaning? Or is seeing a purely sensory event?

References

Als, H. (1977). "The newborn communicates." *Journal of Communication*, 27(2), 66–73.

Als, H. (1982). "Toward a synactive theory of development: promise for the assessment of infant individuality." *Infant Mental Health Journal*, 3(4), 229–243.

Als, H., & Brazelton, T. B. (1981). "A new model of assessing the behavioral organization in preterm and fullterm infants." *Journal of the American Academy of Child Psychiatry*, 20 (2), 239–263.

Buytendijk, F. J. J. (1974). *Prolegomena to an Anthropological Physiology*. Pittsburgh, PA: Duquesne University Press. (Original work published 1965).

Husserl, E. (1989). *Ideas Pertaining to a Pure Phenomenology and to a Phenomenological Philosophy. Second Book: General Introduction to a Pure Phenomenology*. (R. Rojcewicz, A. Schuwer, transl.) Dordrecht: Kluwer. (Original work published 1913).

Ihde, D. (1990). *Technology and the Lifeworld: From Garden to Earth*. Bloomington, IN: Indiana University Press.

Johnson, M. (2007). *The Meaning of the Body: Aesthetics of Human Understanding*. Chicago, IL: University of Chicago Press.

Lang, P. J. (1994). "The varieties of emotional experience: a meditation on James-Lange theory." *Psychological Review*, 101(2), 211–221.

Lean, R. E., Smyser, C. D., & Rogers, C. E. (2017). "Assessment: the newborn." *Child and Adolescent Psychiatric Clinics of North America*, 26(3), 427–440.

Merleau-Ponty, M. (1962). *Phenomenology of Perception*. (C. Smith, transl.) London: Routledge & Kegan Paul Ltd. (Original work published 1945).

Merleau-Ponty, M. (1963). *The Structure of Behavior*. (A. L. Fisher, transl.) Boston, MA: Beacon Press. (Original work published 1942).

Merleau-Ponty, M. (1968). *The Visible and the Invisible*. (A. Lingis, transl.) Evanston, IL: Northwestern University Press. (Original work published 1964).

Nilsson, L. (1973). *Behold Man: A Photographic Journey of Discovery Inside the Body*. Boston, MA: Little, Brown.

Stein, E. (1989). *On the Problem of Empathy*. (W. Stein, transl.) Washington, DC: ICS Publications. (Original work published 1917).

Stern, D. N. (1985). *The Interpersonal World of the Infant: A View from Psychoanalysis and Developmental Psychology*. New York, NY: Basic Books.

Van den Berg, J. H. (1966). *The Psychology of the Sickbed*. New York, NY: Duquesne University Press. (Original work published 1959).

Waters, S. F., West, T. V., & Mendes, W. B. (2014). "Stress contagion: physiological covariation between mothers and infants." *Psychological Science*, 25(4), 934–942.

Zahavi, D. (2014). *Self and Other: Exploring Subjectivity, Empathy, and Shame*. Oxford: Oxford University Press.

5

THE LOOK OF EYE CONTACT

Many parents can recall a moment of being caught in their newborn's gaze. Such moments may occur while preparing to feed, changing a diaper, or quite simply holding. In response to the child's look, a parent may respond with a smile, laugh, or other expression. The interaction may be interrupted, suspended, or merely marked by the briefest moment of pause. The point is that, in such moments, the child is seen in his or her looking; and, the parent experiences being seen.

Yet the gaze of a newborn can be enigmatic. It is not that the child's looking appears peculiar, strange, or abnormal, but instead that the look may touch us, even if we do not know exactly what it says. In a fundamental way, we could say that in the look we sense the otherness of this infant. We realize that he or she is a separate being. And in this experience a sense of otherness of the look prompts us to respond. As Levinas (1969) writes, "The face, preeminently expression, formulates the first word: the signifier arising at the thrust of his sign, as eyes that look at you" (p. 178).

Receiving the look or smile of a baby is different from watching a baby gaze or smile at another person—just as holding a crying baby is quite different from watching someone else hold a crying baby. The experience of the look is observable, yet most touching, when we experience it ourselves. Whether we are touched, stirred, or even agitated from our engagement with a child, there is a definite identifiable experience that may herald our emotional response.

More perplexing than an adult's experience of the look, what might a newborn see? What might constitute a newborn's experience of gazing or staring at its mother's face? What does a newborn's gaze tell us about his or her existence? Merleau-Ponty (1962) would say that experience is rooted in the subjective capacities of our bodies. Yet, we know that newborns differ considerably in their perceptual and cognitive development compared to older children. This is even more true for babies born premature whereby the various body systems

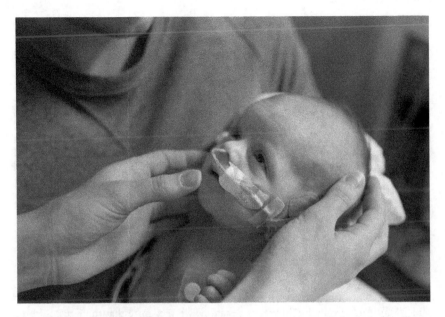

A father and mother cradle their daughter. She stares wide-eyed, body held still. At only a few weeks of age, her gaze is directed towards her mother's face who returns the look in a moment of pause.

themselves are ever so immature in their development. But, we should realize that even preterm children do look. What meaning resides in a newborn's gaze?

The Eyes are Open to the World

How prepared are the eyes to see when a newborn squints at the world, lying against his or her mother's chest? We know that physiologically the eyes are in a constant state of development from the earliest weeks of gestation. Within the womb, clusterings of ectodermal cells within the optic groove of the developing neural tube already form the rudiments of eyes at two weeks gestation (Sadler, 2015). The terms morphogenesis, differentiation, and development describe how the eyes proceed to become anatomically recognizable as sensory apparatuses by four weeks gestation (Sadler, 2015). However, there is no doubt that at this point the eyes are incomplete. Even the eyelids, which seem like little more than flaps of tissue, need to proceed through multiple stages of formation, fusion, development, separation, and maturation (Tawfik et al., 2016).

Yet, the eyes do not need a full 40 weeks of pregnancy gestation to provide some function. When eyelid separation starts at 20 weeks gestation and the lids open in the ensuing weeks, it should not be surprising that the eyes already show signs of activity—blinking or squinting in response to bright light—whether the child has been born early or remains within the womb (Descroix et al., 2015; Petrikovsky et

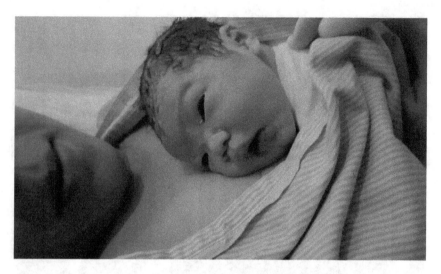

As he lies freshly born, his eyes open to the light of the world.

al., 2003). And already by 30 weeks gestation, we recognize that the fetus, if born, has the capacity to fixate vision on large objects in close proximity (Moore et al., 2015). It would appear that even though the eyes and related structures are incomplete in their development, they are nonetheless active and sensitive, capable of opening to the world. So, we wonder, do they see when they look? What could this seeing be? What visibility composes the world of the newborn?

To see obviously requires more than the functioning of the anatomical parts of the eyes themselves. The eyes need muscles to move, to hold them steady. And of course, the eyes need the integrity of a neural network that includes subcortical and cortical structures of the brain (Mercuri et al., 2007; Ramenghi et al., 2010). We know from behavioral research that visual abilities have a significant relationship with white matter integrity and later emergence of visual cognitive functions (Ricci et al., 2011; Stjerna et al., 2015). The findings of such research suggest that the eyes and neural networks of vision are not simply underdeveloped in preterm and term infants, but already do function as if differently developed compared to those of the older child or adult. The question of 'do they see?' is nuanced in its complexity.

So, Do the Eyes See?

Since the 1960s, visual 'preference' methodologies have been used to understand visual development (Fantz, 1961). In these studies, infants are presented with dissimilar images of pattern, brightness, color, motion, or other factors. If a child spends more time looking at one image than another, it is interpreted that the infant can differentiate the dissimilar features between the images—he or she is

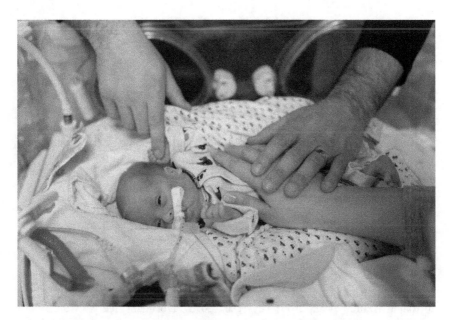

A premature infant lies staring. As parents lay their hands over his body, in time his eyelids will close.

said to 'prefer' that image. From such studies we have learned that the visual field of newborns is narrow compared to the older child, corresponding to the development of retinal vasculature of the eye from the fovea to the periphery (Adolph & Berger, 2015). In comparison, focal length seems to also be relatively fixed such that discrimination between patterns differs depending on how far objects are held from a newborn's face (Adolph & Berger, 2015). However, we need to understand that in studying vision objectively, we ask whether an infant appears to differentiate between visual stimuli rather than whether an infant actually has visual experiences.

Studies of visual impairment and development point to the necessity to constatively question, not just whether newborns behave differentially between two unlike objects, but whether newborns actually have certain visual experiences. For example, despite injury to the occipital cortex, brain injured infants may show the ability to fixate, track, and even show pattern directed gazes in their first weeks to months of life; and yet, these same children may lose these abilities as they mature, becoming observably blind in their sight (Atkinson, 1984; Dubowitz et al., 1986; Martin et al., 1999). Are we certain that the behavior of fixating, tracking, or even showing pattern directed gazes implies a visual experience for the newborn?

Imaging studies, using functional magnetic imaging, show differing patterns of activity in the visual cortex and related subcortical areas in infants compared to adults in response to visual stimuli (Martin et al., 1999). So, if patterns differ, could experiential vision not differ as well? Finally, for infants born premature, specific areas of visual pathway injury have been linked to impairments in visual acuity, contrast sensitivity, color perception, visual fields, motion perception, visual attention, form recognition, and visual memory at later ages in childhood (Chau et al., 2013; Dutton, 2013). But what is vision without sharpness, contrast, form, and so forth? Together such findings introduce the possibility that immaturity, if functionally at all akin to injury, could mean that premature and term newborns have visual experiences that are similar to children and adults with visual pathway injuries. In other words, these findings point to the possibility, if not probability, that visual experiences of newborns may differ from those of adults with intact visual pathways, even if newborns show visual capacities.

We readily talk about vision in isolation, yet in the perceptual world vision is accompanied by smell, taste, touch, sound, and other sense material. Vision is crucial for the development of multi-sensory perception such that visual deprivation effects not only vision development but also the development of other senses (Chen et al., 2017). From studies of congenitally blind individuals who have had their vision restored, we know that vision deprivation between the ages of five months to two years may be associated with an inability to connect vision to touch (Azañón et al., 2017; Ley et al., 2013). Do infants see with their eyes? Or does so-called visual perception also involve touch, taste, and other sensory experience as the eyes open to the world?

And then there is the phenomenon of 'blindsight' that refers to the existence of visual abilities in those who are blind. Despite being unable to describe conscious visual experiences, these blind individuals may display abilities such as object avoidance, direction of motion discrimination, emotional face response, and light source identification (Stoerig & Cowey, 1997; Weiskrantz, 1996). In other words, the blind may experience visual stimuli in a nonvisual manner.

Attention of the Eyes

In the face of behavioral and imaging studies, we may witness infants experiencing the world with their eyes. It has been known for decades that infants tend to fixate on faces. Even in their first minutes and hours after birth, they will direct their gaze at a face over other visual objects (Goren et al., 1975; Johnson & Morton, 1991). The constatation is that the face seems to hold or sustain attention. Relatedly, some have proposed that the newborn brain possesses "innate information concerning the structure of faces" given the newborn's tendency to track significantly more face-like displays when facial features are arranged in a natural way (Morton & Johnson, 1991, p. 170).

Yet, it is not simply that newborns have a visual preference for what is 'face-like,' they seem to look more to faces that have open eyes (Batki et al., 2000). Newborns direct their gaze more at faces that engage with them in gaze (Farroni et al., 2002), and in particular, with those faces that are upright and straight-ahead in orientation (Farroni et al., 2006). Perhaps, these observations correspond to the

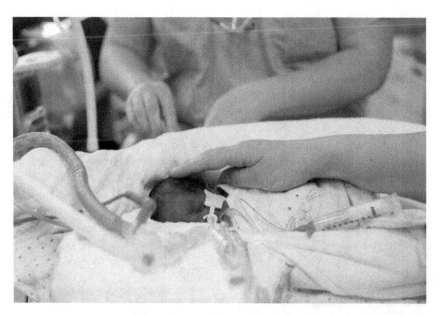

Around him, the world is busy as nurses busily shift around the unit. He appears drowsy with eyes rolling upwards, alternating between convergent and divergent gazes. Every so often, his eyes fix onto his own image reflected in a mirror, then they wander again. A nurse notices his restlessness, and removes the mirror. Now, eyelids close as he begins to drift off to sleep.

newborn looking towards his or her mirrored image. After all, mirrored eyes gaze directly back as the gazing body takes pause. Behavioral researchers do not comment on the significance of the pupils in the gaze of the open eyes. But it is exactly the pupils that are involved in eye contact. When the newborn gazes, then fixates at a face, we see the body quiet, even for the briefest moment, before movement of the eyes or body resumes. Even for the newborn, the look seems to require a response, the demand of which can only be alleviated by removing the mirror.

Behavioral research also tells us that newborns seem to look more at animated than at still faces (Nagy, 2008). And, they seem to look more at a 'new' face rather than a 'known' face—particularly if the 'known' face was previously seen to be fixed, still, or inanimate in expression (Cecchini et al., 2011a). It is as if there is an experience of attention in the look that calls for interaction. As well, it has been observed that the more newborns have visual-imitative interactions with a known face, the more they seem to look at it compared to a novel face (Cecchini et al., 2011a). Studies of contingent visual stimuli have shown that newborns between 12 and 36 hours of age will suck in certain ways to have their mother's face shown compared to another female's face (Walton et al., 1992).

Extensive literature has explored the phenomenon of visual imitation in newborns with the strongest evidence describing newborns having the capacity to imitate facial gestures like tongue protrusion or mouth opening (Meltzoff, 1999; Meltzoff & Moore, 1977). Other behaviors such as lip pursing, head turning, and finger movements have also been reported (Jones, 2017). The constatation is that imitation is the possibility for "absorbing the expressions and gestures of the other into the movements of our own body" (Wider, 1999, p. 204). In such situations, consciousness is bodily without necessarily being self-reflective, meaning the newborn imitates actions without being able to see itself perform (tongue protrusion, mouth opening, or other imitated behaviors). The mirror neuron hypothesis is the prominent theory on infant imitation (Gallese et al., 1996). Mirror neurons are essentially brain cells that are active both in situations of observed action and action performance. It has been speculated, therefore, that newborns possibly experience others' facial expressions or imitated movements as their own (Simpson et al., 2014). Yet, the mirror neuron hypothesis by no means explains all infant behaviors. For example, infants sometimes imitate gestures that were remotely observed, overriding current views (Meltzoff & Moore, 1997).

Looking for Eye Contact

It has long been known that newborns smile during irregular sleep, drowsiness, and alert inactivity: "a slow, gentle, sideward and upward pull of mouth, without rhythmical movements or contraction of other facial muscles" (Wolff, 1959, p. 115).

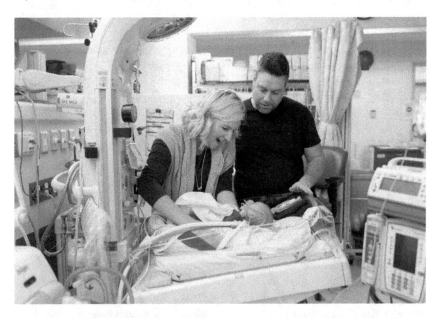

Trying to engage her baby to smile, she moves her face in close, making exaggerated facial expressions. At first, it seems that the baby's gaze simply cannot steady, then the eyes lock in as a smile is born.

And smiling is not simply observed in term newborns but even in extremely premature infants at the cusp of viability (Kawakami et al., 2008) and even within the womb (Kawakami & Yanaihara, 2012; Piontelli, 2010). There is a great deal of literature on smiles observed in newborns suggesting that smiles vary in their meaning (Cecchini et al., 2011b; Dondi et al., 2007; Messinger et al., 1999; 2001; 2002). The more passive smiles of sleep are subtle in their physiognomy with often little more than a raising of the corners of the mouth. In comparison, the perhaps more effortful smiles with an open mouth and raising of the cheeks seem to have meaning related to interaction. As Oster (1978) writes:

Nor do these social smiles resemble reflex like neonatal [sleep] smiles: the brow knitting and prolonged periods of "fascinated" gazing at the caregiver's face that often precede smiling, the variability and complexity of the facial movements accompanying the infant's smiles, and their smooth onset and gradual fading are characteristic of genuine affect expressions, not reflexively elicited responses.

(p. 73).

Such smiles are observed during periods of interactive wakeful exchanges rather than during sleep, a time in which smiles appear to have a different physiognomy (Cecchini et al., 2011a; Lavelli & Fogel, 2005; Messinger & Fogel, 2007). Some have proposed that open-mouth smiles are expressive of joy (Ekman et al., 1990; Messinger et al., 1999). Such smiles can be difficult to elicit in the newborn relative to the infant at a few weeks or months of age (Messinger & Fogel, 2007). Therefore, it is not surprising that many would still say that it is only nearer two months of age that newborns *really* smile. Still we may wonder whether meaningful experiences exist behind infants' facial expressions.

It has been shown by imaging studies that even in a blindsighted individual, portions of the brain respond to eye contact relative to an averted gaze (Burra et al., 2013). It seems that despite lacking a subjective visual experience, there is a response not unlike what is seen in response to emotive facial expressions (Vuilleumier et al., 2003). This observation gives credence to the possibility that eye contact as a phenomenon with or without vision is emotive in its meaning.

We recognize that the first hours of life are a time of activity and alertness. If the awake newborn is unbundled (not held, or otherwise left), he or she will likely move arms and legs, while hands and feet rake the world around. The baby who is not held and unbundled tends to sound agitated or simply cry out. The eyes in such agitated movements lack points of fixation. And even when the newborn is calm, the eyes may fail to steady. Yet, if we are patient enough, and bring our own face into the infant's view, we may find that the gaze steadies to fixate. Even for the premature infant, fixation on the face is a possible response. This means that the fixation may herald more significance than a mere pausing of the eyes. Yet, what is seen?

While we may not be able to actually answer *what* if anything is seen, a different question is whether what is experienced is a sense of contact. While the look is not necessarily a purely visual experience, we may be inclined to look more closely at the newborn him- or herself in gazing. For the infant who smiles while gazing at something or someone, do we not wonder whether experience reflects at the very least contact with a world that may yield some form of contentment. As we watch and look to see what happens in a moment of newborn eye contact we may wonder whether it is simply the eyes that become fixed or whether the whole embodied being of the infant quiets and attends in an ocular touching: the touch of eye contact. The behaviorally bouncing infant body may display an experiential sense of happiness or contentment; the infant body that quiets in the momentary gaze may undergo an experiential sense of touching and being touched.

Concluding Thoughts

While literature on the development of premature newborns is still in its infancy, we recognize that the phenomenon of looking and eye contact continues to change in the months following birth of the term infant. Does the response to visual stimuli constitute a visual experience? It is apparent that infants rely on visual stimuli for development. For example, term infants' vision is monochromatic to red, seemingly a function of light transilluminating hemoglobin within the womb (Clark-Gambelunghe & Clark, 2015); and the development of stereoscopic vision appears to be more dependent on how long it is that a child has been outside of the womb, rather than the child's age in relation to conception (Jandó et al., 2012). For the development of later vision, it seems that infants are resilient in their visual development. Even if their eyes are deprived of vision because of congenital cataract or other obstruction to vision, visual development can still occur if the obstruction is relieved in the first months of life (Lambert & Drack, 1996). Nonetheless, lack of visual input can affect other sensory modalities.

While developmental physiology may help us raise questions regarding sensual experiential possibilities for an infant's visual world, the newborn's meaningful experiences of a visual world is still an enigma. The newborn's eyes may open and be responsive to the world even in the infant who is born premature. Perhaps a phenomenology of the infant gaze requires a different sensitivity to their looking as they make contact with their world. Vision is not simply physiological in its meaning but expresses textures of meaning that we simply fail to 'see' if the gaze is only regarded by what a newborn has the *capacity* to 'see.'

Finally, a discussion of vision as contact turns us back to the language we use to describe the activities, capabilities, and of course presumed experiences of newborns. We need to attend to the language we use to describe a newborn as

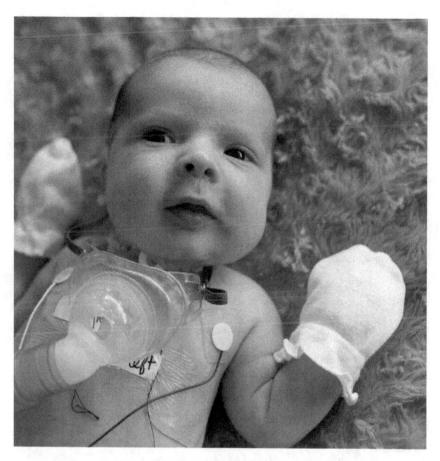

What do his eyes see as he brightens the world with his smile?

making contact with the world. An abstract discourse is not able to make the concrete lived quality of experience visible. Rather a more poetic or pathic language is needed to describe and express the vocative and emotive dimensions of existence. Otherwise, do we really know what we are naming?

References

Adolph, K. E., & Berger, S. E. (2015). "Physical and motor development." In: M. H. Bornstein & M. E. Lamb (eds.), *Developmental Science: An Advanced Textbook, 7th edition*. New York, NY: Psychology Press. pp. 261–333.

Atkinson, J. (1984). "Human visual development over the first six months of life: a review and a hypothesis." *Human Neurobiology*, 3(2), 61–74.

Azañón, E., Camacho, K., Morales, M., & Longo, M. R. (2017). "The sensitive period for tactile remapping does not include early infancy." *Child Development*, 89(4), 1394–1404. doi:10.1111/cdev.12813

Batki, A., Baron-Cohen, S., Wheelwright, S., Connellan, J., & Ahluwalia, J. (2000). "Is there an innate gaze module? Evidence from human neonates." *Infant Behavior and Development*, 23(2), 223–229.

Burra, N., Hervais-Adelman, A., Kerzel, D., Tamietto, M., de Gelder, B., & Pegna, A. J. (2013). "Amygdala activation for eye contact despite complete cortical blindness." *The Journal of Neuroscience*, 33(25), 10483–10489.

Cecchini, M., Baroni, E., Di Vito, C., & Lai, C. (2011b). "Smiling in newborns during communicative wake and active sleep." *Infant Behavior & Development*, 34(3), 417–423.

Cecchini, M., Baroni, E., Di Vito, C., Piccolo, F., & Lai, C. (2011a). "Newborn preference for a new face vs. a previously seen communicative or motionless face." *Infant Behavior & Development*, 34(3), 424–433.

Chau, V., Taylor, M. J., & Miller, S. P. (2013). "Visual function in preterm infants: visualizing the brain to improve prognosis." *Documenta Ophthalmologica*, 127(1), 41–55.

Chen, Y.-C., Lewis, T. L., Shore, D. I., & Maurer, D. (2017). "Early binocular input is critical for development of audiovisual but not visualtactile simultaneity perception." *Current Biology*, 27(4), 583–589.

Clark-Gambelunghe, M. B., & Clark, D. A. (2015). "Sensory development." *Pediatric Clinics of North America*, 62(2), 367–384.

Descroix, E., Charavel, M., Świątkowski, W., & Graff, C. (2015) "Spontaneous eye-blinking rate from pre-term to six-months." *Cogent Psychology* (serial online), 2(1), 1–14.

Dondi, M., Messinger, D., Colle, M., Tabasso, A., Simion, F., Dalla Barba, B., & Fogel, A. (2007). "A new perspective in neonatal smiling: differences between the judgments of expert coders and naive observers." *Infancy*, 12(3), 235–255.

Dubowitz, L. M., Mushin, J., De Vries, L., & Arden, G. B. (1986). "Visual function in the newborn infant: is it cortically mediated?" *Lancet*, 1(8490), 1139–1141.

Dutton, G. N. (2013). "The spectrum of cerebral visual impairment as a sequel to premature birth: an overview." *Documenta Ophthalmologica*, 127(1), 69–78.

Ekman, P., Davidson, R. J., & Friesen, W. V. (1990). "The Duchenne smile: emotional expression and brain physiology II." *Journal of Personality and Social Psychology*, 58(2), 342–353.

Fantz, R. (1961). "The origin of form perception." *Scientific American*, 204, 66–72.

Farroni, T., Menon, E., & Johnson, M. H. (2006). "Factors influencing newborns' preference for faces with eye contact." *Journal of Experimental Child Psychology*, 95(4), 298–308.

Farroni, T., Gergely, C., Simion, F., & Johnson, M. H. (2002). "Eye contact detection in humans from birth." *Proceedings of the National Academy of Sciences*, 99(14), 9603–9605.

Gallese, V., Fadiga, L., Fogassi, L., & Rizzolatti, G. (1996). "Action recognition in the premotor cortex." *Brain*, 119(Pt 2), 593–609.

Goren, C. C., Sarty, M., & Wu, P. Y. K. (1975). "Visual following and pattern discrimination of face-like stimuli by newborn infants." *Pediatrics*, 56(4), 544–549.

Jandó, G., Mikó-Baráth, E., Markó, K., Hollódy, K., Török, B., & Kovacs, I. (2012). "Early-onset binocularity in preterm infants reveals experience-dependent visual development in humans." *Proceedings of the National Academy of Sciences*, 109(27), 11049–11052.

Johnson, M. H., & Morton, J. (1991). *Biology and Cognitive Development: The Case of Face Recognition*. Oxford: Blackwell.

Jones, S. (2017). "Can newborn infants imitate?" *Wiley Interdisciplinary Reviews: Cognitive Science*, 8(1–2), e1410.

Kawakami, F., & Yanaihara, T. (2012). "Smiles in the fetal period." *Infant Behavior and Development*, 35(3), 466–471.

Kawakami, K., Takai-Kawakami, K., Kawakami, F., Tomonaga, M., Suzuki, M., & Shimizu, Y. (2008). "Roots of smile: a preterm neonates' study." *Infant Behavior and Development*, 31(3), 518–522.

Lambert, S. R., & Drack, A. V. (1996). "Infantile cataracts." *Survey of Ophthalmology*, 40(6), 427–458.

Lavelli, M., & Fogel, A. (2005). "Developmental changes in the relationship between the infant's attention and emotion during early face-to-face communication: the 2-month transition." *Developmental Psychology*, 41(1), 265–280.

Levinas, E. (1969). *Totality and Infinity: An Essay on Exteriority*. (A. Lingis, transl.) Pittsburgh, PA: Duquesne University Press. (Original work published 1961).

Ley, P., Bottari, D., Shenoy, B. H., Kekunnaya, R., & Röder, B. (2013). "Partial recovery of visual–spatial remapping of touch after restoring vision in a congenitally blind man." *Neuropsychologia*, 51(6), 1119–1123.

Martin, E., Joeri, P., Loenneker, T., Ekatodramis, D., Vitacco, D., Hennig, J., & Marcar, V. L. (1999). "Visual processing in infants and children studied using functional MRI." *Pediatric Research*, 46(2), 135–140.

Meltzoff, A. N. (1999). "Origins of theory of mind, cognition and communication." *Journal of Communication Disorders*, 32(4), 251–269.

Meltzoff, A. N., & Moore, M. K. (1977). "Imitation of facial and manual gestures by human neonates." *Science*, 198(4312), 75–78.

Meltzoff, A. N., & Moore, M. K. (1997). "Explaining facial imitation: a theoretical model." *Early Development and Parenting*, 6, 179–192.

Mercuri, E., Baranello, G., Romeo, D. M. M., Cesarini, L., & Ricci, D. (2007). "The development of vision." *Early Human Development*, 83(12), 795–800.

Merleau-Ponty, M. (1962). *Phenomenology of Perception*. (C. Smith, transl.) London: Routledge & Kegan Paul Ltd. (Original work published 1945).

MessingerD. S., & Fogel, A. (2007). "The interactive development of social smiling." In: R. V. Kail (ed.), *Advances in Child Development and Behavior*. Cambridge, MA: Elsevier Inc. pp. 327–366.

Messinger, D. S., Fogel, A., & Dickson, K. L. (1999). "What's in a smile?" *Developmental Psychology*, 35(3), 701–708.

Messinger, D. S., Fogel, A., & Dickson, K. L. (2001). "All smiles are positive, but some smiles are more positive." *Developmental Psychology*, 37(5), 642–653.

Messinger, D. S., Dondi, M., Nelson-Goens, G. C., Beghi, A., Fogel, A., & Simion, F. (2002). "How sleeping neonates smile." *Developmental Science*, 5(1), 48–54.

Moore, L. M., Persaud, T. V. N., & Torchia, M. G. (2015). *The Developing Human: Clinical Oriented Embryology*. Philadelphia, PA: Saunders.

Morton, J., & Johnson, M. H. (1991). "CONSPEC and CONLERN: a two-process theory of infant face recognition." *Psychological Review*, 98(2), 164–181.

Nagy, E. (2008). "Innate intersubjectivity: newborns' sensitivity to communication disturbance." *Developmental Psychology*, 44(6), 1779–1784.

Oster, H. (1978). "Facial expression and affect development." In: M. Lewis & L. A. Rosenblum (eds.), *The Development of Affect*. New York, NY: Plenum Press. pp. 43–75.

Petrikovsky, B. M., Kaplan, G., & Holsten, N. (2003). "Eyelid movements in normal human fetuses." *Journal of Clinical Ultrasound*, 31(6), 299–301.

Piontelli, A. (2010) *Development of Normal Fetal Movements: The First 25 Weeks of Gestation.* Milan: Springer-Verlag.

Ramenghi, L. A., Ricci, D., Mercuri, E., Groppo, M., De Carli, A., Ometto, A., Fumagalli, M., Bassi, L., Pisoni, S., Cioni, G., & Mosca, F. (2010). "Visual performance and brain structures in the developing brain of pre-term infants." *Early Human Development*, 86 (Suppl 1), S73–S75.

Ricci, D., Romeo, D. M., Gallini, F., Groppo, M., Cesarini, L., Pisoni, S., Serrao, F., Papacci, P., Contaldo, I., Perrino, F., Brogna, C., Bianco, F., Baranello, G., Sacco, A., Quintiliani, M., Ornetto, A., Cilauro, S., Mosca, F., Romagnoli, C., Romeo, M. G., Cowan, F., Cioni, G., Ramenghi, L., & Mercuri, E. (2011). "Early visual assessment in preterm infants with and without brain lesions: correlation with visual and neurodevelopmental outcome at 12 months." *Early Human Development*, 87(3), 177–182.

Sadler, T. W. (2015). *Langman's Medical Embryology.* Philadelphia, PA: Wolters Kluwer Health.

Simpson, E. A., Murray, L., Paukner, A., & Ferrari, P. F. (2014). "The mirror neuron system as revealed through neonatal imitation: presence from birth, predictive power and evidence of plasticity." *Philosophical Transactions of the Royal Society B: Biological Sciences*, 369, 20130289.

Stjerna, S., Sairanen, V., Gröhn, R., Andersson, S., Metsäranta, M., Lano, A., & Vanhatalo, S. (2015). "Visual fixation in human newborns correlates with extensive white matter networks and predicts long-term neurocognitive development." *The Journal of Neuroscience*, 35(12), 4824–4829.

Stoerig, P., & Cowey, A. (1997). "Blindsight in man and monkey." *Brain*, 120(Pt 3), 535–559.

Tawfik, H. A., Abdulhafez, M. H., Fouad, Y. A., & Dutton, J. J. (2016). "Embryologic and fetal development of the human eyelid." *Ophthalmic Plastic and Reconstructive Surgery*, 32(6), 407–414.

Vuilleumier, P., Armony, J. L., Driver, J., & Dolan, R. J. (2003). "Distinct spatial frequency sensitivities for processing faces and emotional expressions." *Nature Neuroscience*, 6(6), 624–631.

Walton, G. E., Bower, N. J., & Bower, T. G. (1992). "Recognition of familiar faces by newborns." *Infant Behavior and Development*, 15(2), 265–269.

Weiskrantz, L. (1996). "Blindsight revisited." *Current Opinion in Neurobiology*, 6, 215–220.

Wider, K. (1999). "The self and others: imitation in infants and Sartre's analysis of the look." *Continental Philosophy Review*, 32(2), 195–210.

Wolff, P. H. (1959). "Observations on newborn infants." *Psychosomatic Medicine*, 21(2), 110–118.

6

COMING TO TERMS WITH DISTRESS

A fundamental concern of those who practice in neonatal-perinatal medicine is to avoid, alleviate, or at the very least lessen pain, agitation, and other possible experiences of distress. And yet, it is only within the last 30 years that there has been widespread recognition within the medical community that premature and term infants are capable of experiences of pain (Unruh, 1992). Prior to the late 1980s, it was not uncommon that infants would undergo invasive procedures and surgeries without analgesia; newborns were believed to be relatively insensitive to pain (Anand & Hickey, 1987; Scanlon, 1985; Yaster, 1987). Such exposures are now linked with adverse outcomes: physiologic instability (Anand et al., 1987; Grunau et al., 2001), altered stress hormone expression (Anand et al., 1985; Slater et al., 2006), and long-term effects on brain growth and neurodevelopment (Brummelte et al., 2012; Ranger et al., 2013; Smith et al., 2011; Vinall et al., 2014).

Despite advances in clinical care, NICUs remain potentially distressing places for newborns where even the average hospitalized infant is recognized to be subject to multiple painful procedures throughout the day (Carbajal et al., 2008; Johnston et al., 2011; Simons, 2003). It is not simply heelsticks, line insertions, or other technical procedures that may be painful; even a simple activity like a diaper-change may be distressing for a preterm infant (Lyngstad et al., 2014). While avoiding potentially painful, agitating, or otherwise distressing events is the goal, many of these practices remain necessary for the provision of medical care.

When medications are judged necessary, opioids are the most common class of drugs prescribed, although the use of benzodiazepine is also widespread (Borenstein-Levin et al., 2017). Still, there is evolving literature that gives clinicians pause when prescribing medications because analgesic and sedative exposures have been linked to long-term neurodevelopmental outcomes (Anand et al., 1999; 2004; de Graaf et al., 2011; 2013; McPherson & Grunau, 2014; Ranger et al., 2014; Steinhorn et al.,

2015; Zwicker et al., 2016). Without clear evidence of which agent is better, there exists substantial variation in use of narcotic and sedative medications in NICUs (Borenstein-Levin et al., 2017; Carbajal et al., 2015; Johnston et al., 2011). Researchers are also actively engaged in studying all manner of non-pharmacologic measures for their therapeutic benefits: non-nutritive sucking (Carbajal et al., 1999), breast milk (Badiee et al., 2013), breastfeeding (Uga et al., 2008), sugar water (Stevens et al., 2016), acupuncture (Chen et al., 2017), massage (Abdallah et al., 2013), mechanical vibration (McGinnis et al., 2016), gentle touch (Herrington & Chiodo, 2014), holding (Castral et al., 2008), kangaroo care (Johnston et al., 2017), positioning (Kucukoglu et al., 2015), swaddling (Shu et al., 2014), white noise (Kucukoglu et al., 2016), music (Standley, 2001), and maternal voice (Azarmnejad et al., 2015). Still, there is concern that pain is poorly managed in the NICU (Johnston et al., 2011).

The reality is that we know too little about infant pain, agitation, and related disturbing conditions (Fitzgerald, 2015). Although pain and agitation are generally regarded as distinct entities, their behavioral expressions overlap considerably such that health professionals rely heavily on context, intuition, and at times trial-and-error in their attempts to palliate. For example, an infant appearing distressed is most likely considered in pain and therefore treated with an analgesic in the situation of a demonstrable etiology inflicting tissue damage such as trauma, illness, or another event (Broome & Tanzillo, 1990). Conversely, the crying infant who cannot be fed while awaiting surgery may be given a sedative. And yet, can unmet hunger not be painful? Can tissue injury not also lead to unrest? Should possible forms of distress be placed across homogeneous spectrums of pain and agitation? How can the experience of distress be understood in more complex variations and subtle manifestations?

A Distressing Case

Much of the vocabulary describing newborns relates to alertness. A heavily sedated infant neither rouses nor cries in response to stimulation. There are no spontaneous movements and the body appears flaccid or lax. Vital signs are slow or static in response to stimulation. Even breathing may slow to the point of pausing or ceasing in apnea. In contrast, the agitated or pained infant is inconsolable: arching, kicking, constantly awake. Facial expressions are wrinkled or creased as the body is clenched, hands fisted or splayed. Measures of heart rate, respiratory rate, blood pressure, and so forth are increased. Between conditions of sedation and agitation there is a state of 'normality' consisting of arousal with relaxed yet responsive body tone. So, although the baby may cry, he or she can also be calmed; vital signs will vary around an expected baseline.

We might think that the discourse of sedation, agitation, and pain does not require an experiential understanding of what a newborn goes through. Yet, are there not varying dispositions and states of sedation, agitation, and pain? Does the moment of falling asleep in front of the television not differ from the moment of drowsily awakening in the morning? Does the restless agitation experienced from being disoriented in time or place not differ from the pent-up agitation of anger or frustration? Does the pain of a chronic wound not differ from the pain of a sudden prick? Clearly the terms 'sedation,' 'agitation,' and 'pain' do not necessarily name a singular phenomenon. Still, do we not also recognize that there are invariant senses to sedation, agitation, and pain that pervade such varied experiences?

> At only six weeks of age, Maria had already been through multiple cardiac surgeries, invasive procedures, and other interventions for her medical care. Keeping Maria comfortable was difficult and challenging. She was given various analgesic-sedative drugs: morphine, dexmedetomidine, clonidine, and chloral hydrate. Much of the time she was agitated—neither tolerating the gradual reduction nor responding positively to a maintenance or an increase of medication.

Questions were raised: Is Maria in pain? Could she be experiencing withdrawal? Is she getting sick? What could we be missing? All agreed that even considering what Maria had been through, any pain that she could be suffering surely should be improving. Her wounds were healing well and she did not cry out in response to being handled. Her movements were not jittery, nor were there loose stools, nasal congestions, or other signs of medication withdrawal. Possibilities such as a metabolic disturbances, infectious complications, and so forth were all raised; but, her blood work and clinical parameters were reassuring.

Use of pain and agitation assessment tools is a common practice for such children (Carter & Brunkhorst, 2017). These scales use a variety of assessment criteria and descriptors related to observed cry, behavior state, facial expression, extremity tone, and vital sign changes. The most established scales are CRIES—Crying, Requires increased oxygen, Increased vital signs, Expression, Sleeplessness (Krechel & Bildner, 1995), NFCS—the Neonatal Facial Coding System (Grunau & Craig, 1987), NIPS—the Neonatal Infant Pain Score (Lawrence et al., 1993), NPASS—the Neonatal Pain, Agitation, and Sedation Scale (Hummel et al., 2008); and PIPP—the Premature Infant Pain Profile (Stevens et al., 1996). While some of these assessment tools have not been extensively studied, others have received a great deal of attention. They are touted to be valid and reliable scales for assessing preterm and/or full-term newborns. From looking at Maria's scores, it was evident that she should be rated to have pain and/or agitation. And yet, the scores themselves did not tell us what needed to done.

The nurse describes what he sees:

> It seems that, whenever she is awake, she is just agitated. Her suck lacks grasp. She does not really hold a soother in her mouth. Her body movements seem to have no intent and direction. Rather her movements are

composed of squirms, trembles, and kicks regardless of how she is held. Although she looks around and responds, she does not seem to make nor sustain any kind of contact with things. It is like the world around her does not make sense. And when we give her more medications, it gets even worse, unless we absolutely sedate her. I wonder if she ever gets any real sleep. Although there are times in the day when it is a little better, mostly she just appears miserable. Could this be delirium?

The nurse poses an unexpected question. Delirium is an uncommon word in the NICU. Instead, words such as sleepy, tired, alert, hungry, fussy, restless, and so forth are used. And more common clinical terms would be sedation, agitation, and pain.

Diagnosing Delirium

Since ancient times descriptions of what we now call delirium have been accounted for with many different names—sometimes as a symptom and other times as a cluster of symptoms (Adamis et al., 2016). Delirium, from Latin, *delirare* means to literally "deviate from the furrow" (from *de-* 'deviate' and *lira* 'ridge between furrows') (*OED*). In other words, the mental state of delirium is a disturbance from normalcy: to be crazy, deranged, silly, rave, or quite simply, 'out of one's wits' (Lewis et al., 1879).

In contemporary medicine, delirium formally represents an umbrella construct, adopted to overcome varied terminology used to describe disturbances in consciousness (European Delirium Association & American Delirium Society, 2014). In the third version of the *Diagnostic and Statistical Manual of Mental Disorders* (DSM-III), delirium is identified as a 'clouding of consciousness' (American Psychiatric Association, 1981; European Delirium Association & American Delirium Society, 2014). In subsequent versions of the DSM, the term consciousness is linked to the construct of attention, driven by the recognition that 'consciousness' is difficult to assess objectively (American Psychiatric Association, 1987, 1994, 2000). Someone who is disturbed in consciousness is difficult to engage in attention. In the most recent version of DSM-V the core feature of delirium is: "Disturbance in attention (i.e. reduced ability to direct, focus, sustain, and shift attention) and awareness (reduced orientation to the environment)" although delirium remains de facto a disturbance in consciousness (American Psychiatric Association, 2013, p. 596).

In pediatric and adult critical care communities, delirium is not only a common diagnosis, but also frequently passed over or missed (Hatherill & Flisher, 2010). An observer makes a diagnosis of delirium based on a perceived difficulty in engaging and sustaining awareness and attention, noting that actions are lacking purpose or betray unawareness, and on perceived problems with communication or altered activity. Yet, the diagnostic term 'delirium' is relatively absent from the NICU with only a few published cases describing its existence in early infancy

(Groves et al., 2016). As such, it would certainly not be unexpected for even an experienced neonatologist, nurse, or other practitioner working in a NICU to look puzzled in response to the question of delirium.

Is the lack of attention to the possible diagnosis of delirium in the NICU a problem? Many of the factors usually associated with delirium exist in the NICU: use of analgesic-sedative medications, loss of routines connected with feeding and/or sleep, and complicated medical conditions necessitating interruptions in physical contact between caregivers and their patients. How could it be that infants hospitalized in intensive care would not experience delirium? Yet, if a newborn's primal conscious is in some way unique, underdeveloped, or undifferentiated, can the newborn actually experience delirium? Or perhaps might a newborn's existence in some way already be characterized by delirium? Vice versa, when we describe children or adults as experiencing delirium, are they living through a reality that is more akin or somehow resembling that of a newborn?

The problem is that we cannot possibly know whether a newborn suffers from perceptual experiences such as hallucinations or delusions as described in children and adults with delirium diagnoses (Andersson et al., 2002; Duppils & Wikblad, 2007; Fagerberg & Jönhagen, 2002; Grover et al., 2009; Leentjens et al., 2008; McCurren & Cronin, 2003; Schofield, 1997; Stenwall et al., 2008; Turkel et al., 2006). Nor can we know whether newborns have reported experiences of disreality, dream-like states, or other experiential sensations of a clouding of consciousness (Andersson et al., 2002; McCurren & Cronin, 2003). While we may witness an infant on sedative, analgesic, or otherwise neurologically active medications appear 'out of it,' staring blankly into space or exhibiting rapidly shifting gazes, we cannot know *what* he or she experiences. Rather, when his or her body moves without seeming direction, 'out of sync' to what is offered, we may be only able to say that he or she is quite simply not him- or herself. A soother may be offered yet the mouth does not grasp or seems only able to gasp at it. Or an infant may appear agitated no matter what is offered: food, touch, or some other comfort. Objectively we may say that the newborn appears disturbed in his or her attention and awareness, but recognizing our desire for objectivity may place in abeyance the possible subjectivity of the infant's experience. So, if we name a newborn as delirious, we are limited to suggest that their world-experience is changed.

From reports by adults, what is seen, heard, smelt, or otherwise experienced in delirium can be variable in its meaningfulness. A hallucination may be recounted as intensely emotional with feelings of anxiety or fear (Andersson et al., 2002; Duppils & Wikblad, 2007; Fagerberg & Jönhagen, 2002; Laitinen, 1996; McCurren & Cronin, 2003; Schofield, 1997; Stenwall et al., 2008). Other times, hallucinations are described as pleasurable (Andersson et al., 2002; Duppils & Wikblad, 2007; Schofield, 1997). And for some adults the experience of delirium while enigmatic may be marked by a "disinterested perplexity" (O'Malley et al., 2008, p. 225). It would seem that the emotionality of a delirium experience is in part commensurate with *what* is experienced in a moment of delirium. But distress is not an invariant feature of delirium.

Ought we then to wonder whether infants without signs of distress may nevertheless be subject to perceptual disturbances that are similar to delirium? Are newborns capable of having lived through experiences of pleasure or confusion if their perception is altered? When a newborn tries to suck at the breast and no milk is to be had, what does he or she experience? Or, when a newborn shakes, extends, or otherwise arches his or her body without any semblance of being held what then is being experienced? Watching a baby flush, shake, or cry out, it is hard to constatively conclude that such events do not have significance for a baby. Yet, how can we know that a baby is delirious when attempting to feed, and yet it cannot? Does the experience of delirium vary from baby to baby? Could it be associated with cognitive elements or development?

Focusing on Interaction and Empathy

The baby in the opening vignette was six weeks old when the question of delirium was raised. Other published reports of delirium include infants as young as four weeks of age (Groves et al., 2016). If indeed we are comfortable assigning 'delirium' to a newborn, what meaning resides in the term? Developmentally we could say that to apply the term 'delirium' necessitates a constatative recognition that newborns have unified and organized perceptions that can be disturbed. We have a certain awareness that such disturbances are possible even though the precise subjectivity of these events cannot be ascertained.

For the above child, we actually considered the diagnosis of delirium. We adopted the Cornell Assessment of Pediatric Delirium (Traube et al., 2014) such that the bedside assessment focus shifted to considering Maria's actions as expressive of disordered perception using descriptive anchors such as eye contact, purposefulness of actions, state of behavior, response to soothing measures, and other expected interactions. Treatment decisions were focused on weaning off medications that were thought to contribute to disturbances of perception rather than escalate medications to combat pain or agitation. And yet, to assume the presentation of delirium required empathic understanding and a qualitative questioning: a "focused human attention and sincere commitment to the infant's comfort" (Anand & Hall, 2008, p. 826). Raising the question of delirium could not have been possible if medical care was simply given procedurally, mechanistically, or otherwise distanced from a concern for possible experiential meaning for Maria.

Although we cannot know whether the term 'delirium' is truly appropriate to apply to a newborn, we need to question what is at stake if we do not raise such diagnostic questions? The application of a term such as delirium to the world of the infant is more than a philosophical affair but rather expresses an effort to value possible infant experiences, to consider what we are actually treating. It shows a concern for newborns to be comfortable. As well, the discourse of delirium may express an abiding interest into an infant's possible perception of the world.

In contrast, we need to ask what do we risk when we use technical neologisms or other terms drained of recognized sensuality such as 'disorganized behavior,' 'co-regulation,' or 'neonatal encephalopathy' in our conversations about the wellbeing of newborns. We need to ask what is lost if we rely exclusively on objective criteria, concepts, and rating scales to diagnose and assess an infant's wellbeing. The question is not whether pain or agitation scales should or should not be routinely used in making decisions about weaning or starting medications—after all these tools have the potential to promote quality professional healthcare. Yet, we need to remember that such tools are relatively devoid of the richness afforded by the unique descriptions of interactions between infants and caregivers. How was his last feed? How did she settle after the procedure? What is she like when she is awake? These are appropriate questions to ask when making decisions regarding the use of analgesic-sedative medications, particularly if we want to attend not simply to measured values but also to the meaningfulness of our patients' possible experience. Assessment scales ultimately reflect an adult's objective understanding of pain, agitation, delirium, and so forth—which is in fact also subjective (i.e. reflecting an adult observer's subjectivity). Therefore, if used, it would seem prudent that NICU staff have a clear understanding of the limits of such tools and that they always ensure to look holistically at a child.

Concluding Thoughts

So in the end, although we may be unable to say whether newborns experience delirium, perhaps we ought to wonder whether they can. And perhaps more pointedly such wondering may benefit from a qualitative understanding. We need to be sensitive to the meanings inherent in the language of sedation, agitation, pain, and delirium, recognizing that such understandings for the newborn (and especially for the premature newborn) will always be partial and incomplete.

Clearly advances are being made in the empirical studies of infant pain, agitation, and other possible experiences of distress. It is relatively recent that we now have evidence that shows that the cortex of even premature babies is activated in response to potentially painful stimulation (Bartocci et al., 2006; Slater et al., 2006). Similarly, electroencephalographic studies show that there is a temporal and spatial pattern of brain activity that follows noxious stimuli in the newborn and that changes with maturation (Fabrizi et al., 2011; Slater et al., 2010a; 2010b; Verriotis et al., 2015). Research also points to the need to be cognizant that outward appearances of distress may vary with illness, maturity, and other factors (Gibbins et al., 2008; Johnston & Stevens, 1996). Perceived distressing behaviors do not necessarily correspond to distressing experiences (Fitzgerald, 2015).

Most research has focused on acute procedural pain with limited attention to recurrent, prolonged, or chronic pain (Ranger et al., 2007). So it is possible that

NICU infants suffer pain, agitation, and other possible experiences of distress without outward appearances. Similarly, it is possible that supposed therapeutic interventions only mask the expression of distress without actually alleviating pain, agitation, or other experiences of distress if they only act on subcortical mediating structures (Fitzgerald, 2015). Thus, we need to ensure as health professionals that when we consider whether to wean, increase, or otherwise adjust medications for comfort that we remain open in our understanding of the inner life of the hospitalized infant. We constantly need to ask about the meaning of the observations, anecdotes, and narratives that point to possible experiences in our newborn patients.

References

Abdallah, B., Badr, L. K., & Hawwari, M. (2013). "The efficacy of massage on short and long term outcomes in preterm infants." *Infant Behavior and Development*, 36(4), 662–669.

Adamis, D., Treloar, A., Martin, F. C., & Macdonald, A. J. D. (2016). "A brief review of the history of delirium as a mental disorder." *History of Psychiatry*, 18(4), 459–469.

American Psychiatric Association. (1981). *Diagnostic and Statistical Manual of Mental Disorders, 3rd Edition*. Washington, DC: American Psychiatric Association.

American Psychiatric Association. (1987). *Diagnostic and Statistical Manual of Mental Disorders: DSM-IIIR*. Washington, DC: American Psychiatric Association.

American Psychiatric Association. (1994). *Diagnostic and Statistical Manual of Mental Disorders: DSM-IV*. Washington, DC: American Psychiatric Association.

American Psychiatric Association. (2000). *Diagnostic and Statistical Manual of Mental Disorders: DSM-IV-TR*. Washington, DC: American Psychiatric Association.

American Psychiatric Association. (2013). *Diagnostic and Statistical Manual of Mental Disorders: DSM-5*. Arlington, VA: American Psychiatric Association.

Anand, K. J., & Hickey, P. R. (1987). "Pain and its effects in the human neonate and fetus." *New England Journal of Medicine*, 317(21), 1321–1329.

Anand, K. J., Sippel, W. G., & Aynsley-Green, A. (1987). "Randomised trial of fentanyl anasethesia in preterm babies undergoing surgery: effects on the stress response." *Lancet*, 329(8527), 243–248.

Anand, K. J., Brown, M. J., Bloom, S. R., & Aynsley-Green, A. (1985). "Studies on the hormonal regulation of fuel metabolism in the human newborn infant undergoing anaesthesia and surgery." *Hormone Research*, 22(1–2), 115–128.

Anand, K. J., Barton, B. A., McIntosh, N., Lagercrantz, H., Pelausa, E., Young, T. E., & Vasa, R. (1999). "Analgesia and sedation in preterm neonates who require ventilator support: results from the NOPAIN trial: neonatal outcome and prolonged analgesia in neonates." *Archives of Pediatrics & Adolescent Medicine*, 153(4), 331–338.

Anand, K. J., Hall, R. W., Desai, N., Shephard, B., Bergqvist, L. L., Young, T. E., Boyle, E. M., Carbajal, R., Bhutani, V. K., Moore, M. B., Kronsberg, S. S., & Barton, B. A.; NEOPAIN Trial Investigators Group. (2004). "Effects of morphine analgesia in ventilated preterm neonates: primary outcomes from the NEOPAIN randomised trial." *Lancet*, 363(9422), 1673–1682.

Anand, K. J. S., & Hall, R. W. (2008). "Love, pain, and intensive care." *Pediatrics*, 121(4), 825–827.

Andersson, E. M., Hallberg, I. R., Norberg, A., & Edberg, A. K. (2002). "The meaning of acute confusional state from the perspective of elderly patients." *International Journal of Geriatric Psychiatric*, 17(7), 652–663.

Azarmnejad, E., Sarhangi, F., Javadi, M., & Rejeh, N. (2015). "The effect of mother's voice on arterial blood sampling induced pain in neonates hospitalized in neonate intensive care unit." *Global Journal of Health Science*, 7(6), 198–204.

Badiee, Z., Asghari, M., & Mohammadizadeh, M. (2013). "The calming effect of maternal breast milk odor on premature infants." *Pediatrics and Neonatology*, 54(5), 322–325.

Bartocci, M., Bergqvist, L. L., Lagercrantz, H., & Anand, K. J. (2006). "Pain activates cortical areas in the preterm newborn brain." *PAIN*, 122(1–2), 109–117.

Borenstein-Levin, L., Synnes, A., Grunau, R. E., Miller, S. P., Yoon, E. W., & Shah, P. S.; Canadian Neonatal Network Investigators. (2017). "Narcotics and sedative use in preterm neonates." *Journal of Pediatrics*, 180, 92–98.

Broome, M. E., & Tanzillo, H. (1990). "Differentiating between pain and agitation in premature neonates." *Journal of Perinatal Neonatal Nursing*, 4(1), 53–62.

Brummelte, S., Grunau, R. E., Chau, V., Poskitt, K. J., Brant, R., Vinall, J., Gover, A., Synnes, A. R., & Miller, S. P. (2012). "Procedural pain and brain development in premature newborns." *Annals of Neurology*, 71(3), 385–396.

Carbajal, R., Chauvet, X., Couderc, S., & Olivier-Martin, M. (1999). "Randomised trial of analgesic effects of sucrose, glucose, and pacifiers in term neonates." *British Medical Journal*, 319(7222), 1393–1397.

Carbajal, R., Rousset, A., Danan, C., Coquery, S., Nolent, P., Ducrocq, S., Saizou, C., Lapillonne, A., Granier, M., Durand, P., Lenclen, R., Coursol, A., Hubert, P., de Saint Blanquat, L., Boëlle, P. Y., Annequin, D., Cimerman, P., Anand, K. J., & Bréart, G. (2008). "Epidemiology and treatment of painful procedures in neonates in intensive care units." *JAMA*, 300(1), 60–70.

Carbajal, R., Eriksson, M., Courtois, E., Boyle, E., Avila-Alvarez, A., Andersen, R. D., Sarafidis, K., Polkki, T., Matos, C., Lago, P., Papadouri, T., Montalto, S. A., Ilmoja, M. L., Simon, S., Tameliene, R., van Overmeire, B., Berger, A., Dobrzanska, A., Schroth, M., Bergqvist, L., Lagercrantz, H., & Anand, K. J.; EUROPAIN Survey Working Group. (2015). "Sedation and analgesia practices in neonatal intensive care units (EUROPAIN): results from a prospective cohort study." *The Lancet Respiratory Medicine*, 3(10), 796–812.

Carter, B. S., & Brunkhorst, J. (2017). "Neonatal pain management." *Seminars in Perinatology*, 41(2), 111–116.

Castral, T. C., Warnock, F., Leite, A. M., Haas, V. J., & Scochi, C. G. (2008). "The effects of skin-to-skin contact during acute pain in preterm newborns." *European Journal of Pain*, 12(4), 464–471.

Chen, K. L., Quah-Smith, I., Schmölzer, G. M., Niemtzow, R., & Oei, J. L. (2017). "Acupuncture in the neonatal intensive care unit-using ancient medicine to help today's babies: a review." *Journal of Perinatology*, 37(7), 749–756.

De Graaf, J., van Lingen, R. A., Valkenburg, A. J., Weisglas-Kuperus, N., Groot Jebbink, L., Wijnberg-Williams, B., Anand, K. J., Tibboel, D., & van Dijk, M. (2013). "Does neonatal morphine use affect neuropsychological outcomes at 8 to 9 years of age?" *PAIN*, 154(3), 449–458.

De Graaf, J., van Lingen, R. A., Simons, S. H., Anand, K. J., Duivenvoorden, H. J., Weisglas-Kuperus, N., Roofhooft, D. W., Groot Jebbink, L. J., Veenstra, R. R., Tibboel, D., & van Dijk, M. (2011). "Long-term effects of routine morphine infusion in mechanically ventilated neonates on children's functioning: five year follow-up of a randomized controlled trial." *PAIN*, 152(6), 1391–1397.

Duppils, G. S., & Wikblad, K. (2007). "Patients' experiences of being delirious." *Journal of Clinical Nursing*, 16(5), 810–818.

European Delirium Association & American Delirium Society. (2014). "The DSM-5 criteria, level of arousal and delirium diagnosis: inclusiveness is safer." *BMC Medicine*, 12, 141.

Fabrizi, L., Slater, R., Worley, A., Meek, J., Boyd, S., Olhede, S., & Fitzgerald, M. (2011). "A shift in sensory processing that enables the developing human brain to discriminate touch from pain." *Current Biology*, 21(18), 1552–1558.

Fagerberg, I., & Jönhagen, M. E. (2002). "Temporary confusion: a fearful experience." *Journal of Psychiatric and Mental Health Nursing*, 9(3), 339–346.

Fitzgerald, M. (2015). "What do we really know about newborn infant pain?" *Experimental Physiology*, 100(12), 1451–1457.

Gibbins, S., Stevens, B., McGrath, P. J., Yamada, J., Beyene, J., Breau, L., Camfield, C., Finley, A., Franck, L., Johnston, C., Howlett, A., McKeever, P., O'Brien, K., & Ohlsson, A. (2008). "Comparison of pain responses in infants of different gestational ages." *Neonatology*, 93(1), 10–18.

Grover, S., Malhotra, S., Bharadwaj, R., Bn, S., & KumarS. (2009). "Delirium in children and adolescents." *International Journal of Psychiatry in Medicine*, 39(2), 179–187.

Groves, A., Traube, C., & Silver, G. (2016). "Detection and management of delirium in the neonatal unit: a case series." *Pediatrics*, 137(3), e20153369.

Grunau, R. V. E., & Craig, K. D. (1987). "Pain expression in neonates: facial action and cry." *PAIN*, 28(3), 395–410.

Grunau, R. E., Oberlander, T. F., Whitfield, M. F., Fitzgerald, C., & Lee, S. K. (2001). "Demographic and therapeutic determinants of pain reactivity in very low birth weight neonates at 32 weeks' postconceptional age." *Pediatrics*, 107(1), 105–112.

Hatherill, S., & Flisher, A. J. (2010). "Delirium in children and adolescents: a systematic review of the literature." *Journal of Psychosomatic Research*, 68(4), 337–344.

Herrington, C. J., & Chiodo, L. M. (2014). "Human touch effectively and safely reduces pain in the newborn intensive care unit." *Pain Management Nursing*, 15(1), 107–115.

Hummel, P., Puchalski, M., Creech, S. D., & Weiss, M. G. (2008). "Clinical reliability and validity of the N-PASS: neonatal pain, agitation and sedation scale with prolonged pain." *Journal of Perinatology*, 28(1), 55–60.

Johnston, C., Barrington, K. J., Taddio, A., Carbajal, R., & Filion, F. (2011). "Pain in Canadian NICUs: have we improved over the past 12 years?" *Clinical Journal of Pain*, 27 (3), 225–232.

Johnston, C., Campbell-Yeo, M., Disher, T., Benoit, B., Fernandes, A., Streiner, D., Inglis, D., & Zee, R. (2017). "Skin-to-skin care for procedural pain in neonates." *Cochrane Database of Systematic Reviews*, 2, CD008435.

Johnston, C. C., & Stevens, B. J. (1996). "Experience in a neonatal intensive care unit affects pain response." *Pediatrics*, 98(5), 925–930.

Krechel, S. W., & Bildner, J. (1995). "CRIES: a new neonatal postoperative pain measurement score. Initial testing of validity and reliability." *Pediatric Anesthesia*, 5(1), 53–61.

Kucukoglu, S., Kurt, S., & Aytekin, A. (2015). "The effect of the facilitated tucking position in reducing vaccination-induced pain in newborns." *Italian Journal of Pediatrics*, 41, 61.

Kucukoglu, S., Aytekin, A., Celebioglu, A., Celebi, A., Caner, I., & Maden, R. (2016). "Effect of white noise in relieving vaccination pain in premature infants." *Pain Management Nursing*, 17(6), 392–400.

Laitinen, H. (1996). "Patients' experience of confusion in the intensive care unit following cardiac surgery." *Intensive and Critical Care Nursing*, 12(2), 79–83.

Lawrence, J., Alcock, D., McGrath, P., Kay, J., MacMurray, S. B., & Dulberg, C. (1993). "The development of a tool to assess neonatal pain." *Neonatal Network*, 12(6), 59–66.

Leentjens, A. F. G., Schieveld, J. N. M., Leonard, M., Lousberg, R., Verhey, F. R. J., & Maegher, D. J. (2008). "A comparison of the phenomenology of pediatric, adult, and geriatric delirium." *Journal of Psychosomatic Research*, 64(2), 219–223.

Lewis, C. T., Short, C., & Andrews, E. A. (1879) *Harpers' Latin Dictionary: A New Latin Dictionary Founded on the Translation of Freund's Latin-German Lexicon*, Ed. By E. A Andrews, LL. D. New York, NY: American Book Company.

Lyngstad, L. T., Tandberg, B. S., Storm, H., Ekeberg, B. L., & Moen, A. (2014). "Does skin-to-skin contact reduce stress during diaper change in preterm infants?" *Early Human Development*, 90(4), 169–172.

McCurren, C., & Cronin, S. N. (2003). "Delirium: elders tell their stories and guide nursing practice." *MEDSURG Nursing*, 12(5), 318–423.

McGinnis, K., Murray, E., Cherven, B., McCracken, C., & Travers, C. (2016). "Effect of vibration on pain response to heel lance." *Advances in Neonatal Care*, 16(6), 439–448.

McPherson, C., & Grunau, R. E. (2014). "Neonatal pain control and neurologic effects of anesthetics and sedatives in preterm infants." *Clinics in Perinatology*, 41(1), 209–227.

O'Malley, G., Leonard, M., Maegher, D., & O'Keeffe, S. T. (2008). "The delirium experience: a review." *Journal of Psychosomatic Research*, 65(3), 223–228.

Ranger, M., Johnston, C. C., & Anand, K. J. S. (2007). "Current controversies regarding pain assessment in neonates." *Seminars in Perinatology*, 31(5), 283–288.

Ranger, M., Synnes, A. R., Vinall, J., & Grunau, R. E. (2014). "Internalizing behaviours in school-age children born very preterm are predicted by neonatal pain and morphine exposure." *European Journal of Pain*, 18(6), 844–852.

Ranger, M., Chau, C. M., Garg, A., Woodward, T. S., Beg, M. F., Bjornson, B., Poskitt, K., Fitzpatrick, K., Synnes, A. R., Miller, S. P., & Grunau, R. E. (2013). "Neonatal pain-related stress predicts cortical thickness at age 7 years in children born very preterm." *PLoS ONE*, 8(10), e76702.

Scanlon J. (1985). "Barbarism in the nursery." *Perinatal Press*, 9(7), 103–104.

Schofield, I. (1997). "A small exploratory study of the reaction of older people to an episode of delirium." *Journal of Advanced Nursing*, 25(5), 942–952.

Shu, S. H., Lee, Y. L., Hayter, M., & Wang, R. H. (2014). "Efficacy of swaddling and heel warming on pain response to heel stick in neonates: a randomized control trial." *Journal of Clinical Nursing*, 23(21–22), 3107–3114.

Simons, S. H., van Dijk, M., Anand, K. S., Roofthooft, D., van Lingen, R. A., & Tibboel, D. (2003). "Do we still hurt newborn babies? A prospective study of procedural pain and analgesia in neonates." *Archives of Pediatrics & Adolescent Medicine*, 157(11), 1058–1064.

Slater, R., Fabrizi, L., Worley, A., Meek, J., Boyd, S., & Fitzgerald, M. (2010a). "Premature infants display increased noxious evoked neuronal activity in the brain compared to healthy age-matched term-born infants." *NeuroImage*, 52(2), 583–589.

Slater, R., Cantarella, A., Gallella, S., Worley, A., Boyd, S., Meek, J., & Fitzgerald, M. (2006). "Cortical pain responses in human infants." *Journal of Neuroscience*, 26(14), 3662–3666.

Slater, R., Worley, A., Fabrizi, L., Roberts, S., Meek, J., Boyd, S., & Fitzgerald, M. (2010b). "Evoked potentials generated by noxious stimulation in the human infant brain." *European Journal of Pain*, 14(3), 321–326.

Smith, G. C., Gutovich, J., Smyser, C., Pineda, R., Newnham, C., Tjoeng, T. H., Vavasseur, C., Wallendorf, M., Neil, J., & Inder, T. (2011). "Neonatal intensive care unit stress is associated with brain development in preterm infants." *Annals of Neurology*, 70(4), 541–549.

Standley, J. M. (2001). "Music therapy for the neonate." *Newborn and Infant Nursing Reviews*, 1(4), 211–216.

Steinhorn, R., McPherson, C., Anderson, P. J., Neil, J., Doyle, L. W., & Inder, T. (2015). "Neonatal morphine exposure in very preterm infants—cerebral development and outcomes." *Journal of Pediatrics*, 166(5), 1200–1207.

Stenwall, E., Jonhagen, M. E., Sandberg, J., & Fagerberg, I. (2008). "The older patient's experience of encountering professional carers and close relatives during an acute confusional state: an interview study." *International Journal of Nursing Studies*, 45(11), 1577–1585.

Stevens, B., Johnston, C., Petryshen, P., & Taddio, A. (1996). "Premature Infant Pain Profile: development and initial validation." *Clinical Journal of Pain*, 12(1), 13–22.

Stevens, B., Yamada, J., Ohlsson, A.Haliburton, S., & Shorkey, A. (2016). "Sucrose for analgesia in newborn infants undergoing painful procedures." *Cochrane Database of Systematic Reviews*, 7, CD001069.

Traube, C., Silver, G., Kearney, J., Patel, A., Atkinson, T. M., Yoon, M. J., Halpert, S., Augenstein, J., Sickles, L. E., Li, C., & Greenwald, B. (2014). "Cornell assessment of pediatric delirium: a valid, rapid, observational tool for screening delirium in the PICU." *Critical Care Medicine*, 42(3), 656–663.

Turkel, S. B., Trzepacz, P. T., & Tavare, C. J. (2006). "Comparing symptoms of delirium in adults and children." *Psychosomatics*, 47(4), 320–324.

Uga, E., Candriella, M., Perino, A., Alloni, V., Angilella, G., Trada, M., Ziliotto, A. M., Rossi, M. B., Tozzini, D., Tripaldi, C., Vaglio, M., Grossi, L., Allen, M., & Provera, S. (2008). "Heel lance in newborn during breastfeeding: an evaluation of analgesic effect of this procedure." *Italian Journal of Pediatrics*, 34(1), 3.

Unruh, A. M. (1992). "Voices from the past: ancient views of pain in childhood." *Clinical Journal of Pain*, 8(3), 247–254.

Verriotis, M., Fabrizi, L., Lee, A., Ledwidge, S., Meek, J., & Fitzgerald, M. (2015). "Cortical activity evoked by inoculation needle prick in infants up to one-year old." *PAIN*, 156(2), 222–230.

Vinall, J., Miller, S. P., Bjornson, B. H., Fitzpatrick, K. P., Poskitt, K. J., Brant, R., Synnes, A. R., Cepeda, I. L., & Grunau, R. E. (2014). "Invasive procedures in preterm children: brain and cognitive development at school age." *Pediatrics*, 133(3), 412–421.

Yaster, M. (1987). "Analgesia and anesthesia in neonates." *Journal of Pediatrics*, 111(3), 394–395.

Zwicker, J. G., Miller, S. P., Grunau, R. E., Chau, V., Brant, R., Studholme, C., Lui, M., Synnes, A., Poskitt, K. J., Stiver, M. L., & Tam, E. W. (2016). "Smaller cerebellar growth and poorer neurodevelopmental outcomes in very preterm infants exposed to neonatal morphine." *Journal of Pediatrics*, 172, 81–87.e2.

7

SUCKLING AND THE BEING OF THE NEWBORN

Mother and child lie skin-to-skin. Their bodies rise and fall with each breath. The baby's shrugging of the shoulders, twisting of the trunk, and pushing of the legs leverage movement. As the body curves and contorts, a cheek may brush against the mother's skin: the mouth opens, combing the skin. When a free arm flails, extends and flexes, it swipes or perhaps grips at air. And if a hand is momentarily caught on the lips, we witness a chewing, mashing suck, before the hand is released to flail. The baby's mouth remains open. Thrust up, the head lifts and rises momentarily above the skin, eyes open and close. The body is active. When the corner of the mouth meets the nipple, the lips spread to receive it. Breath is drawn in. One, then another, and finally a succession of sucks as a slow steady rhythm of the suckling begins.

For a long time, many healthcare professionals assumed that the brain and nervous system structures of newborns were too immature to permit meaningful perception (Unruh, 1992). The sucking and feeding of an infant was regarded as inborn, innate, or instinctive (Barlow et al., 2001; McGowan et al., 1991; Walker, 1990). From such assumption, the activity of feeding a baby was reduced to reading an infant's cues and providing matching nursing responses.

The subjective life of young infants was felt to be impervious to our understanding, and therefore pointless to try to consider of import. And so, the pursuit of a subjectivity of the newborn was dismissed, deemed outside of legitimate inquiry on both methodological and theoretical grounds. But as Daniel Stern (1985) reminds us, it is precisely the experiential world of the newborn that we need to consider:

> Yet that is at the heart of what we really want and need to know. What we imagine infant experience to be like shapes our notions of who the infant

is ... determine how we, as parents, respond to our own infants, and ultimately they shape our views of human nature.

(p. 4)

Empirical researchers have discovered complex neural, cognitive, and motor developments in the fetus and newborn. In response, the medical professional is realizing the importance of considering the sensory experiences of infants who require medical care (Pineda et al., 2017). Although such researchers have explored the benefits of providing sensory interventions, there has been limited scholarly attention given to promoting possible experiential meanings of such experiences. In other words, now we face questions of an entirely different order. What could newborn experiences be like? How does the infant experience or make sense of the world he or she is born into? How do the sense and meanings the child experience contribute to their growth?

Although we have all been infants, our early days of supposed simply eating, sleeping, and pooping are too distant and remote for memory. And perhaps, in part, the reason we cannot consciously recall such early childhood experiences, is that they were never lived through as distinct events. This does not mean that the newborn exists as simply a repertoire of patterned behavior. Instead, perhaps what is there is simply a life where consciousness is fundamentally primal (Husserl, 1991). Some believe that for the newborn, contemplative self-awareness is nascent—just now coming into active life in the exploration of the world (Trevarthen & Aitken, 2003). Others believe that newborns may only be conscious in the 'point mode' of the 'here and now,' but otherwise void of reflexive subjectivity (Donaldson, 1993).

Neurobiological and psychological researchers have explored the possibility of newborn consciousness (Lagercrantz, 2014). Such researchers generally look for evidence that a baby meets defined theoretical models of consciousness including such criteria as awareness of the body, of one-self, and of the outside world (Velmans & Schneider, 2007). The dialogue surrounding this research while having the potential of clarifying what constitutes an infant's perceptual experience, and how it might resemble adult experience, has largely remained fixated on proving or disproving consciousness models (Lagercrantz & Changeux, 2010; Rochat, 2003). Philosophical researchers, such as Claude Romano, see experience as an allied yet distinct concept of consciousness. Experience is the primal structure of being-in-the-world, which includes a being's subjective capacities as well as the given circumstances in which these abilities are exercised (Romano, 2015, p. 456).

A phenomenology of suckling may be a crucial key for examining the conscious sensuality of newborns. A suckling is an infant who is "at the breast or is unweaned" (*OED*). I use the term 'suckling' to express a concern for not just the act of keep as sucking but also the sense of the being of the newborn who is dependent on the world encountered in sucking. In providing neonatal intensive care, there are all manner of activities that are necessarily undertaken in the medical care of a newborn with processes, challenges, and consequences for the suckling.

The Sensual Beginnings of Suckling

Sucking begins in the womb. A child can actually be born with blisters on his or her hands, forearms, or elsewhere from vigorous prenatal sucking (Monteagudo & León-Muiños, 2010). Research indicates that active mouth opening begins at 7–9 weeks gestation, swallowing of amniotic fluid happens at 12–14 weeks gestation, and sucking occurs at 15–18 weeks gestation (Achiron et al., 1997; D'Elia et al., 2001; Horimoto et al., 1989; Miller et al., 2003; Yan et al., 2006). These sucking movements initially appear spontaneous, without inducement, such that it is not clear whether in their early forms sucking behaviors are volitional, compelled, and accompanied by certain semblances of perception (de Vries et al., 1988).

Perception would appear to begin as the sensory systems reach sufficient maturity to respond to the environment, whether it is fetal or neonatal (Streri et al., 2013). Amniotic fluid is the medium of fetal existence within the womb. The fluid surrounding and soaking the fetus is in continuous contact with the nose, lips, and tongue of the fetus. In the womb, the fetus swallows this liquid whenever sucking movements occur (Miller et al., 2003). Amniotic fluid bears flavor— based on what is ingested (fruit, vegetables, spices) or inhaled (tobacco, perfumes) by the mother (Mennella, 2007). Olfaction of the amniotic fluid is the taste and smell of the womb for the fetal infant.

It is not simply amniotic fluid that fills a fetus' mouth: a hand, a part of the arm, or even the umbilical cord may be introduced into the mouth (de Vries et al., 1982; Hepper et al., 1991; Kurjak et al., 2003; Piontelli, 2010). From as early as 19 weeks gestation, a fetus may be observed to open or close its mouth in relation to self-touching movements of the face (Humphrey, 1970; Myowa-Yamakoshi & Takeshita, 2006). And as the fetus develops from 24–36 weeks gestation, it appears to increasingly touch its lower face and mouth (Reissland et al., 2014). However, there do appear variations in the overall frequency and to some respect the patterns of which fetuses touch their head and other body parts during development. Still, when watching these movements it is easy to imagine that the fetus exists in a state of conscious sensuality—a consciousness that is at the very least composed of experiencing (Sartre, 1956, p. 320).

The mouth itself is touch—lips may press against each other in contact just as the tongue may explore the interiority of the mouth. These bodily parts are highly sensual: dense with sensory receptors with corresponding cortical representation (Schoenfeld et al., 2004). Piaget (1950) did not have access to contemporary fetal research during his classic writings, otherwise he might have extended his sensorimotor theory of learning to the womb. There is research evidence for the perceptual existence of an oral sense of the wombed child: the amniotic fluid appears to be remembered by the newborn after birth

(Schaal et al., 1998; Varendi & Porter, 2001). Hand movements to the mouth appear coordinated from birth depending on the specifics of situations (Blass et al., 1989; Rochat et al., 1988). As well, hand-mouth movements initially appear body-oriented and only after the second month become object-oriented (Rochat, 1993). Still, there is mystery as to the nature of primal consciousness and meaning-impressions of this primary perception.

We know the fetus and newborn have various sensual capacities (olfactory, tactile, auditory, etc.), and research shows that there are perceptual links between sensory modalities for newborns, and presumably also for the fetus (Sann & Streri, 2007; Slater et al., 1997). Experiences are not simply synthetic, involving each of the primary senses, but likely consist of (amodal or multimodal) textured senses that transcend any single sensory modality (Johnson, 2007; Stern, 1985). It may be that experiences lack relation to a single sense, or that various senses may be experienced simultaneously.

Despite our difficulties in qualifying this primal perception, it would perhaps be reasonable to constatate that for the fetus and newborn the elements of suckling encompass sensuality from both the constant (taste-smell of the amniotic fluid) and the variable (touch of hands and arms) textures of experience. Indeed, the taste-smell of amniotic fluid is recognized by the infant after birth (Schaal et al., 1998). And with respect to variable sensations following birth, and even just prior to birth, fetuses may be observed to open their mouths more frequently just before they touch themselves and in response to self-touches of the face (Amiel-Tison & Grenier, 1980; Reissland et al., 2014).

The Familiarity of Suckling

At first glance, birth presents the newborn as individuated, and new to the world (Merleau-Ponty, 2010). Clamping the umbilical cord severs the physical connection of mother and child. Outside of the womb, the newborn may be looked upon in his or her entirety; held or even carried away from the mother. But, a newborn who stirs to awaken may attempt to root in expectation, or cry beyond consolations at soothing. As we return the baby to the mother to feed, we realize that the umbilical cord was only part of the connection.

One of the most visually striking observations of the first minutes of life is the ability of a newborn—if left quietly on a mother's abdomen after birth—to crawl up to her breast, find the nipple, and begin to suckle (Widström et al., 1987).

> If the infant is dried thoroughly and placed on her abdomen and not taken from the mother for the next 60 minutes, the infant begins a five-part sequence. For the first 30 minutes, the newborn rests and looks at his mother intermittently. Between 30 and 40 minutes, lip-smacking and mouthing of the fingers begin, followed by an outpouring of saliva onto the infant's chin. Then the infant begins to inch forward with his legs to push strongly into the

mother's lower abdomen. When he reaches the tip of the sternum, he bounces his head into her chest. While moving up, he often turns his head from side to side. As he comes close to the nipple, he opens his mouth widely and, after several attempts, makes a perfect placement on the areola of the nipple.

(Klaus, 1998, p. 1244)

Born into a cold world, marked by foreign smells and tastes, the breast crawl perhaps heralds the return to what was usual or familiar. The areola of the breast has a perceptively high temperature relative to the surrounding tissue (Zanardo & Straface, 2015). And the vibrations of maternal heartbeat are nowhere more easily felt than against her chest. The colostrum, milk, and even the sweat that exudes from the maternal breasts share the odors and tastes of amniotic fluid (Mennella, 2007). The breast crawl is fragile in its integrity in that it is easily disrupted by other activities or events that may interrupt the contact of newborn and mother (Righard & Blade, 1994).

Husserl (1991) has posited how temporal moments of conscious existence are primordially given as waves in a stream of (pre)conscious experiencing such that experience is caught up in a primal structure of protention–primal impression–retention. The metaphor of waves speaks not only to the differentiated nature of experience—the infant is not overwhelmed by seamless, unstructured sensations—but also to the temporal nature of lived experience itself. The primal impression is the moment of the *now* which has always just-elapsed into a momentary past (retention) yet also anticipates in a more or less indefinite way the next moment of the future (protention). For example, without such a temporal structure we could not experience continuity such as musical melody because individual notes would be given singularly, lacking melodic and rhythmic structure and cohesion. This notion of primordial conscious experiencing locates nicely within our contemporary, cognitive understanding of the newborn. Operant conditioning and naturalistic experiments have shown that newborns are not only conscious of temporal sensations (such as prosody, melodic contour of speech, language, and music), but also retain such sensations in memory (Cooper & Aslin, 1989; DeCasper & Spence, 1986; Granier-Deferre et al., 2011; Hepper, 1988).

According to Casey (2000) "memory of taste (and of smell, closely associated with it) perdures because of its capacity to permeate one's entire sensibility" (p. 253). Research evidences that newborns orient to the fullness of this remembered impressional sense such that if a breast is cleansed, the newborn will track to the opposite, more potent side (Varendi et al., 1994). While we cannot possibly know the exact texture of how taste infuses a newborn's sensibility, watching a baby enact the breast crawl reveals the pluri-sensorial situation of suckling, and memory of suckling, involving touch, vision, and hearing in addition to olfaction. The capacity for memory appears to be present early in development, from about

30 weeks gestation, with formed memories persisting to at least six weeks after delivery (Granier-Deferre et al., 2011).

There is an obvious difference between retaining and protending the tones that have just sounded and are about to sound, and remembering a past holiday or looking forward to the next vacation. Whereas the two latter are full-blown memorable experiences that presuppose the primal work of the retention and the protention, the protention and retention are dependent moments of any occurrent experience. In other words, protention and retention do not provide us with additional intentional objects, but with a (pre)consciousness of the temporal horizon of the present object. Whereas recollection and expectation are, at least to some extent, subject to our will, that is, whereas they are intentional acts that we can initiate ourselves, we cannot stop having retentions and protentions. They are passive processes, preconscious experiences that take place without our active contribution (Zahavi, 2005, p. 58).

Although experience would appear to be a requisite for reflection—for (pre) consciousness to be made an object of reflection as self-reflection—we do not know whether a newborn actually has the capacity to have reflective memory experiences. We can only cautiously wonder whether the movements of the breast crawl express an encountering of the traces of a world as the traces have been encountered before in the womb. Carefully, in supposing preconscious familiarity we must navigate related notions of belonging, comfort, and intimacy that we cannot claim to fully understand to exist in the fetus, though we might claim these qualities for the newborn.

The Intersubjectivity of Suckling

Simms suggests that a newborn's experiencing of the world reflects a directedness that transcends the physical margins of its corporeality: "*that is already pre-figured in one's own body*" (Simms, 2008, p. 26). We detect such directed intentionality in the newborn's relative fixed visual acuity whereby the mother's face seems to be given clarity to vision from the child's position of being held. Significantly, the newborn's open mouth matches in shape to the mother's nipple.

In order for a newborn to be able to feed, he or she needs to be able to orally grasp and express from the nipple. From a physiological perspective, suction corresponds to the generation of negative intraoral pressure to draw milk into the mouth. The draw is the result from the increase of the volume of the oral cavity, complemented by closure of the nasal passages by the soft palate and the tight seal of the lips to prevent air inflow (Lau et al., 2000). Expression consists of compression and stripping of the tongue against the hard palate to eject milk into mouth (Waterland et al., 1998). While suction and expression develop in concert, as far as rhythm and amplitude of each component, it would appear that maturation of expression occurs before that of suction, given that the presence of suction is rarely observed alone (Amaizu et al., 2008; Lau, 2016).

So-called primitive reflexes may be used to elicit the oral movements of suckling (Woolridge, 1986). Stroking of the cheek or mouth may lead the newborn to move its head in steadily, decreasing, rooting arcs until an object is found, and touching the roof the newborn's mouth elicits sucking. These behaviors speak to the manner in which a newborn's body already presupposes the appearance of the world: intentionally adapted and ready to respond to the presence of the mother's breast (Simms, 2008). Yet, even if parts of these behaviors are reflexive, shared with other mammals, Merleau-Ponty (1963) reminds us that experience is not separate to behavior; experience is conditioned by how our body is enmeshed within the world. So even if suckling encompasses a repertoire of reflexive behaviors, the activity of feeding is not necessarily without perceptual form.

We can imagine that even a newborn's suckling has a 'subjective' feel to it. Husserl (2001) differentiates between the intentional matter of the experience (that which is sucked) and the subjective intentional quality of an experience (suckling in itself), recognizing that these dimensions cannot be wholly separated. While we need to be cautious that physiological likenesses do not ensconce that which might differ between mouthing, latching, sucking, and other seemingly related oral phenomena, we may wonder what is generally the subjective intentional quality of suckling? In the context of adult consciousness, the philosopher Dan Zahavi (2005) points out that there is always a quality of mineness, "first-personal givenness" to all experience (p. 124). For example, when I experience hunger I know that this experience is mine and not someone else's. Applied to the newborn, might that mean that the baby's experience of suckling is also felt as his or her own? Mineness is the term that Zahavi uses to describe the sense of subjective self that accompanies all personal experience. Many years earlier, the philosopher Jean-Paul Sartre (1991) had famously argued that in everyday life we do not experience a *self* at all. He gave the example of running for the bus. When running to catch a bus there is no self, said Sartre. We are simply running for the bus. Only when we later tell someone, "I had to run for the bus" does the self (in the form of the 'I') suddenly appear. Thus, the 'I' is an objectification, according to Sartre. It suddenly appears when reflecting on the self. But Zahavi contests this view of the self. He argues that there is always a subsidiary awareness of self to all human experience. So we may wonder, if this existential sense of self accompanies all subjective experience then the newborn too may have a subsidiary self, however primal it may still be.

And yet, Merleau-Ponty (1968) writes of an "anonymous visibility" that fundamentally inhabits us in our earliest of beginnings (p. 142). The visible margins of the body, the appearance of individuation, are illusions of a perception that is syncretic.

The solitude from which we emerge to intersubjective life is not that of the monad. It is only the haze of an anonymous life that separates us from being; and the barrier between us and others is impalpable. If there is a break, it is not between me and the other person; it is between a primordial generality we are intermingled in and the precise system, myself–the others. What "precedes" intersubjective life cannot be numerically distinguished from it, precisely because at this level there is neither individuation nor numerical distinction.

(Merleau-Ponty, 1964, p. 174)

Behavioral studies show that newborn infants mirror oral gestures within hours of birth, such as mouth opening, tongue protrusion, lip widening, lip pursing, as well as complex facial expressions (Field et al., 1982; 1983; Meltzoff & Moore, 1977; 1983; 1994; 1997; Nagy et al., 2005; 2007; Reissland, 1988). A mirror neuron hypothesis has been proposed: "observed actions are understood in terms of one's own action programmes" (Simpson et al., 2014, p. 1). Said differently, and perhaps taken more radically, these observations beg us to consider whether a newborn may actually experience an other's action as his or her own.

Although a shared perceptual existence may in some sense be possible, research does provide constatative evidence that a newborn does at least to some degree or in some manner differentiate its own body from that of another. For example, newborns show increased rooting in response to external-tactile stimulation compared to self-tactile stimulation (Rochat & Hespos, 1997). Still we may wonder what is the sense of mineness of newborn subjective-consciousness to its own body? Does newborn perception entail in part a shared existence without differentiation? Does a newborn experience suckling as of its own being and volition?

Feeding, of course, requires more than active generation and expression of suction. Milk must be passed from the mouth to the stomach. Initially, milk is held in the mouth, aided by a pinching together of the posterior tongue and soft palate to prevent premature fluid spilling into the pharynx and deeper airway (Lau et al., 2000). Thereafter, anterograde peristalsis from the pharynx to the upper esophageal sphincter clears fluid from the mouth. And finally, food passes to the stomach by the coordinated effects of the upper esophageal sphincter, esophageal body, and lower esophageal sphincter. Regardless of the satiety of a newborn, these latter activities occur automatically if provoked.

It is clear from research, and popular literature, that successful feeding is in part baby-led, following an infant's cues (Shloim et al., 2016). From a behavioral perspective, rooting and sucking vary depending on the activity of the child and the timing of recent feeding. The classic observations of Kaye (1967) describe newborns showing an increase in observable sucking behaviors in the time lead-ing up to a feed, particularly if they are awake. And immediately following a feed, these behaviors decrease in frequency until again welling up later. Perhaps, suckling involves aspects of deprivation, desire, or drive in a basic sense—appetite and hunger—an expectation or wanting to be able to suck (Kuperus, 2007). This expectation and wanting are signs of self-sense or agency in the infant's subjectivity. As Zahavi (2005) writes, "the newborn does not have to master the words and concepts 'pain,' 'hunger,' 'frustration,' and 'mine,' in order to feel the mineness of the pain, the hunger, and the frustration" (p. 204).

So, we may wonder to what extent is suckling volitional given that the supposed 'reflexes' for rooting and sucking are not consistently reflexive. The constational suggestion is that an infant cannot necessarily be coaxed to latch onto a nipple simply by putting it within his or her mouth—as in the case of swallowing which is largely autonomic, and cannot be held back. In other words, there appears to be the possibility for experiential dimensions to suckling that could transcend an infant's subjectivity. So perhaps more pointed than questioning whether suckling is reflexive is asking whether a newborn's perception is limited by the margins of his or her body. Does a newborn realize the world beyond his or her body as wholly other to his or her own?

Engaged in Suckling

Established terms in the medical literature are nutritive and non-nutritive sucking, corresponding to whether significant milk is ingested or not. Nutritive sucking occurs at one cycle per second and non-nutritive sucking at two cycles per second with differences in speed presumably due to the need to coordinate swallowing larger volumes of milk obtained from nutritive sucking with breathing (Koenig et al., 1990; Wolff, 1968). Non-nutritive sucking has long been used as a dependent variable in infant perception experiments (Kaye, 1967). In these studies, infants are generally exposed to various stimuli with researchers watching for changes in sucking patterns as evidence of perceptual-discrimination and memory-learning. For example, the experiments by DeCasper and Fifer (1980) revealed that newborns suck more in response to recordings of their mothers' voices compared to those of strangers' voices. This experiment provides evidence for a newborn's capacity to discriminate between voices, proof that its own mother's voice has been retained in memory. Similar studies have shown the ability to discriminate and recognize other sense material such as the odor of amniotic fluid (Varendi et al., 1996), meters or vocal patterns of stories (DeCasper & Spence, 1986), and so forth. The phenomenological question is, what is experientially given in these moments?

In the moment of suckling a baby is flexed with arms and legs held inwards as if contained. Hands may appear to be tight in grip, stretching through motions of opening and closing, or simply held extended in fixed position. As an onlooker, we could say that the posture of the baby in feeding, particularly against the mother's chest, is fetal in position. As a feed progresses most infants will settle, and some will progress to slumber. In contrast, the physiognomy of crying is completely different. In crying, the legs and arms may flail and even shake. The baby's head is straight or hyperextended with mouth open rather than active in grasp. While the cry is perhaps the expression of an unsettling we may speculate that, in contrast, suckling expresses a settling into a soothing sensuality.

Those who take care of infants surely recognize the calming power of suckling in that a crying baby can be calmed by given the opportunity to suck (Rovee & Levin, 1966). It is not simply that the baby can be calmed in the act of sucking, but rather that the baby is engaged, occupied, and engrossed: "captured by the joy of the sensations" (Buytendijk, 1953, p. 11). It is thus perhaps not surprising that even the familiar odors associated with suckling (amniotic fluid and milk) can have a calming effect on a newborn (Rattaz et al., 2005; Varendi et al., 1998). In suckling a newborn can be submerged to the world such that providing an infant with an opportunity to suck reduces the appearance of pain associated with medical procedures even when no milk or sugar is provided (Carbajal et al., 1999; Mathai et al., 2006; Thakkar et al., 2016). It is as if the body *in the suck* is rendered partially insensate. Perhaps the Heideggerian (1995) description of the "undetermined I" fits here whereby the newborn is so absorbed in an activity that the senses themselves are quelled (p. 143).

Suckling offers the possibility for re-encountering familiar or novel sensual textures. We recognize that the newborn when deprived of 'normal sucking opportunities' will spend more time sucking their fingers or other materials (Levy, 1928). Suckling is obviously part of the being of a newborn engaged in the world. Yet, suckling also has its limits. Following feeding (or the sucking of something novel for some period of time), the physiognomy of suckling changes with more frequent occurrences of rest periods, decreased amplitude of suckling decreased or even released pressure, disorganization of the sucking response, and difficulty in acceptance of the nipple (Jensen, 1932). So, it would appear that the constatation is that suckling may allow an infant to slip into sleep from a sensuality of familiarity, engagement, and fulfillment—yet also prepare an infant to encounter newness and novelty of the world.

Complicating Suckling

When babies are born significantly premature or have congenital anomalies, transitional problems, or other medical issues necessitating time in the NICU, it may simply be necessary to hold off on oral feeding for lack of physiological readiness (Jackson et al., 2016). For example, babies born before 28 weeks gestation, while having the ability to suck and swallow, do so in an uncoordinated fashion, such that they are unable to satisfactorily orally feed; while babies with significant lung disease may be unable to safely coordinate feeding with rapid breathing (Koenig et al., 1990; Mathew et al., 1985; Miller & DiFiore, 1995; Rosen et al., 1984). A phenomenology of suckling raises the question what is at stake when suckling is abjured.

The premature or ill newborn inhabits a different oral world than the healthy newborn. In the NICU, the baby's mouth is usually the necessary entry for breathing and feeding tubes. Silastic devices may be needed for days, weeks, or even months such that the texture of oral sensuality becomes in part the constant contact with plastic tubes, adhesive tapes, or other material-devices. The mouth may be intermittently suctioned for secretions. Hands may be bundled in mittens to discourage direct contact between hands and mouth for fear of dislocating necessary medical equipment. We do not really understand the nature of sensuality of such experiences. Researchers have shown that infants who have been cared for in a NICU, and presumably exposed to odorous disinfectant and detergents, show different cerebral hemodynamic responses compared to the exposure of seemingly pleasant flavors like vanilla and colostrum (Bartocci et al., 2000, 2001).

Even if nutrition is provided by intravenous line, without a full stomach, some infants require analgesic or sedative medication to settle. Often when feeds can be introduced, the mouth is bypassed such that it is not unusual to see newborns sucking on breathing or feeding tubes. The question is, what is the relationship of caregiver and child for oral feeding to occur? What is the relational quality of the activity of feeding for the newborn when the mouth or other part of the body no longer are in contact with the mother? While filling an infant's stomach by means of a feeding tube and offering a soother may be enough to calm some infants, others may continue to be unsettled. The oral world for the NICU newborn may unfortunately be relatively existentially detached from the mother, as the needed medical technologies and the designed environment of the NICU itself, may compromise or disrupt parental connection (van Manen, 2012).

These issues aside, there are possibilities for other forms of contact with the lips for premature and ill infants (Pineda et al., 2017). Even intubated infants with central lines on multiple medications can be placed skin-to-skin in contact with their parent in what is affectionately known as kangaroo care (Chan et al., 2016). Colostrum may be painted or instilled into a baby's mouth, and even if not quite ready to feed, a baby may be brought to explore (by way of the mouth) a mother's pumped breast (Lee et al., 2015). Research points to the value of contact for parent and child, and of at least offering a baby an opportunity to suck when tube feeds are given (Foster et al., 2016; Pinelli & Symington, 2005). Such acts give the baby the possibility for recovering the traces of womb world through the mouth.

For premature or ill infants, and even for some healthy newborns, the first oral feed is often a bottle. Breastfeeding seems to require a certain maturity in the form of a competent and strong suck, and it may be challenging for a baby to retain a mother's nipple within his or her mouth (Lau et al., 2007). There is also a medical attraction to the bottle because the clinical team can calculate exactly a baby's intake to monitor feeding as either successful or not, depending on the measure of the volume of feeds obtained. There is a great deal of pressure for babies to achieve oral feeds because once a baby is orally feeding, he or she generally will be able to be discharged home (Eichenwald et al., 2001; Schanler et al., 1999). Prolonged oral feeding difficulties increase medical costs and potential long-term oral feeding aversion and further increase maternal stress as mother–infant reunion is delayed (Lau & Hurst, 1999; Lau et al., 2007; Mason et al., 2005; Melnyk et al., 2008; et al., 1993).

So, to aid attainment of oral feeding it is not unusual to see nurses or parents essentially expressing milk into the back of an infant's mouth such that it is reflexively swallowed with seemingly little suck or expression demonstrated on the part of the infant. The significant issue related to this practice is that the baby cannot help but swallow when fed far back into the pharynx. But what memories are forming for these newborns? Casey (2000) describes body memory as the sedimentation of actions, "past in the body" to inform "present bodily actions" (pp. 149, 150). From this perspective, oral aversion expresses the present of a past forceful feeding. The concern is not simply that the older infant will not take the bottle, but that this newborn had been subjected to repetitive episodes of force-feeding; perhaps more aptly described as force-swallowing. The potential problem is that traumatic body memories may fragment the lived body—breaking it down into uncoordinated parts, incapable of the appropriate action (Casey, 2000). Without deeply rooted positive memories for effective feeding and the possibility of traumatic memories, there is also the concern that these infants may actually grow up not developing in their suckling. Such may be the result when *quantity* of feeding replaces *quality* of feeding as a measure of success.

It is crucial for those who work in the NICU to look not just at how much an infant feeds, but also how an infant appears when he or she feeds. Caregivers should constantly consider how they facilitate newborns to experience the world sensually with their mouths, limbs, and skin. The question is not simply is a child 'ready to feed' as far as safety, but also whether we can support the child to have familiar, intentional, and engaging experiences of feeding, recognizing that sensuality is not simply at the mouth but also involves the infant's bodily being-in-the-world. In other words, watching only for adverse events on trying to feed a baby is not adequate to show readiness to feed. Readiness can only be established by looking for cues of infant interest, inclination, and willingness.

Concluding Thoughts

While the issue of consciousness and subjectivity of the newborn remains an enigma, we do need to remember that from a developmental perspective the newborn will accrue experiences from and into whatever beginning of life he or she is born. We need to constantly ask what beginning we are giving children who are cared for in a NICU. In whatever modalities it may be conceived or understood, the world has incarnate, perceptual, and emotional meaning for the child and his or her others. And the meaning the world has for others affects the meaning it will have for the newborn (Zahavi, 2005).

References

Achiron, R., Ben Arie, A., Gabbay, U., Mashiach, S., Rotstein, Z., & Lipitz, S. (1997). "Development of the fetal tongue between 14 and 26 weeks of gestation: in utero ultrasonographic measurements." *Ultrasound in Obstetrics & Gynecology*, 9(1), 39–41.

Amaizu, N., Shulman, R., Schanler, R., & Lau, C. (2008). "Maturation of oral feeding skills in preterm infants." *Acta Paediatrica*, 97(1), 61–67.

Amiel-Tison, C., & Grenier, A. (1980). *Evaluation Neurologique du Nouveau-né et du Nourrisson*. Paris: Masson.

Barlow, S. M., Dusick, A., Finan, D. S., Coltart, S., & Biswas, A. (2001). "Mechanically evoked perioral reflexes in premature and term infants." *Brain Research*, 899(1–2), 251–254.

Bartocci, M., Winberg, J., Papendieck, G., Mustica, T., Serra, G., & Lagercrantz, H. (2001). "Cerebral hemodynamic response to unpleasant odors in the preterm newborn measured by near-infrared spectroscopy." *Pediatric Research*, 50(3), 324–330.

Bartocci, M., Winberg, J., Ruggiero, C., Bergqvist, L. L., Serra, G., & Lagercrantz, H. (2000). "Activation of olfactory cortex in newborn infants after odor stimulation: a functional near-infrared spectroscopy study." *Pediatric Research*, 48(1), 18–23.

Blass, E. M., Fillion, T. J., Rochat, P., Hoffmeyer, L. B., & Metzger, M. A. (1989). "Sensorimotor and motivational determinants of hand-mouth coordination in 1–3-day-old human infants." *Developmental Psychology*, 25(6), 963–975.

Buytendijk, F. J. J. (1953). "Experienced freedom and moral freedom in the child's consciousness." *Educational Theory*, 3(1), 1–13.

Carbajal, R., Chauvet, X., Couderc, S., & Olivier-Martin, M. (1999). "Randomised trial of analgesic effects of sucrose, glucose, and pacifiers in term neonates." *British Medical Journal*, 319(7222), 1393–1397.

Casey, E. S. (2000). *Remembering: A Phenomenological Study*. Bloomington, IN: Indiana University Press.

Chan, G. J., Valsangkar, B., Kajeepeta, S., Boundy, E. O., & Wall, S. (2016). "What is kangaroo mother care? Systematic review of the literature." *Journal of Global Health*, 6(1), 010701.

Cooper, R. P., & Aslin, R. N. (1989). "The language environment of the young infant: implications for early perceptual development." *Canadian Journal of Psychology*, 43(2), 247–265.

D'Elia, A., Pighetti, M., Moccia, G., & Santangelo, N. (2001). "Spontaneous motor activity in normal fetuses." *Early Human Development*, 65(2), 139–147.

De Vries, J. I., Visser, G. H., & Prechtl, H. F. (1982). "The emergence of fetal behaviour: I. Qualitative aspects." *Early Human Development*, 7(4), 301–322.

De Vries, J. I. P., Visser, G. H. A., & Prechtl, H. F. R. (1988). "The emergence of fetal behaviour. III. Individual differences and consistencies." *Early Human Development*, 16(1), 85–103.

DeCasper, A. J., & Fifer, W. P. (1980). "Of human bonding: newborns prefer their mothers' voices." *Science*, 208(4448), 1174–1176.

DeCasper, A. J., & Spence, M. J. (1986). "Prenatal maternal speech influences newborn's perception of speech sounds." *Infant Behavior and Development*, 9(2), 133–150.

Donaldson, M. (1993). *Human Minds: An Exploration*. London: Allen Lane, The Penguin Press.

Eichenwald, E. C., Blackwell, M., Lloyd, J. S., Tran, T., Wilker, R. E., & Richardson, D. K. (2001). "Inter-neonatal intensive care unit variation in discharge timing: influence of apnea and feeding management." *Pediatrics*, 108(4), 928–933.

Field, T. M., Woodson, R., Greenberg, R., & Cohen, D. (1982). "Discrimination and imitation of facial expressions by neonates." *Science*, 218(4568), 179–181.

Field, T. M., Woodson, R., Cohen, D., Greenberg, R., Garcia, R., & Collins, K. (1983). "Discrimination and imitation of facial expressions by term and preterm neonates." *Infant Behavior and Development*, 6(4), 485–489.

Foster, J. P., Psaila, K., & Patterson, T. (2016). "Non-nutritive sucking for increasing physiologic stability and nutrition in preterm infants." *Cochrane Database of Systematic Reviews*, 10, CD001071.

Granier-Deferre, C., Bassereau, S., Ribeiro, A., Jacquet, A.-Y., & DeCasper, A. J. (2011). "A melodic contour repeatedly experienced by human near-term fetuses elicits a profound cardiac reaction one month after birth." *PLoS ONE*, 6(2), e17304.

Heidegger, M. (1995) *The Fundamental Concepts of Metaphysics: World, Finitude, Solitude.* (W. McNeill, N. Walker, transl.) Bloomington, IN: Indiana University Press. (Original work published 1983).

Hepper, P. G. (1988). "Fetal 'soap' addiction." *Lancet*, 1(8598), 1347–1348.

Hepper, P. G., Shahidullah, S., & White, R. (1991). "Handedness in the human fetuses." *Neuropsychologia*, 29(11), 1107–1111.

Horimoto, N., Koyanagi, T., Nagata, S., Nakahara, H., & Nakano, H. (1989). "Concurrence of mouthing movement and rapid eye movement/non-rapid eye movement phases with advance in gestation of the human fetus." *American Journal of Obstetrics & Gynecology*, 161(2), 344–351.

Humphrey, T. (1970). "Reflex activity in the oral and facial area of the human fetus." In: J. F. Bosma (ed.), *Second Symposium on Oral Sensation and Perception*. Springfield, IL: Charles C. Thomas. pp. 195–233.

Husserl, E. (1991). *On the Phenomenology of the Consciousness of Internal Time (1893–1917).* (J. B. Brough, transl.) Dordrecht: Kluwer Academic. (Original work published 1966).

Husserl, E. (2001). *Logical Investigations, Volume 1.* (J. N. Findlay, transl.) Oxon: Routledge. (Original work published 1900/1901).

Jackson, B. N., Kelly, B. N., McCann, C. M., & Purdy, S. C. (2016). "Predictors of the time to attain full oral feeding in late preterm infants." *Acta Paediatrica*, 105(1), e1–6.

Jensen, K. (1932). "Differential reactions to taste and temperature stimuli in newborn infants." *Genetic Psychological Monographs*, 12(5–6), 363–479.

Johnson, M. (2007). *The Meaning of the Body: Aesthetics of Human Understanding*. Chicago, IL: University of Chicago Press.

Kaye, H. (1967). "Infant sucking behavior and its modification." *Advances in Child Development and Behavior*, 3, 1–52.

Klaus, M. (1998). "Mother and infant: early emotional ties." *Pediatrics*, 102(sup E1), 1244–1246.

Koenig, J. S., Davies, A. M., & Thach, B. T. (1990). "Coordination of breathing, sucking, and swallowing during bottle feedings in human infants." *Journal of Applied Physiology*, 69(5), 1623–1629.

Kuperus, G. (2007). "Attunement, deprivation, and drive: Heidegger and animality." In: C. Lotz & C. Painter (eds.), *Phenomenology and the Non-Human Animal: At the Limits of Experience*. Dordrecht: Sage. pp. 13–27.

Kurjak, A., Azumendi, G., Vecek, N., Kupesic, S., Solak, M., Varga, D., & Chervenak, F. (2003). "Fetal hand movements and facial expression in normal pregnancy studied by four-dimensional sonography." *Journal of Perinatal Medicine*, 31(6), 496–508.

Lagercrantz, H. (2014). "The emergence of consciousness: science and ethics." *Seminars of Fetal and Neonatal Medicine*, 19(5), 300–305.

Lagercrantz, H., & Changeux, J. P. (2010). "Basic consciousness of the newborn." *Seminars in Perinatology*, 34(3), 201–206.

Lau, C. (2016). "Development of infant oral feeding skills: what do we know?" *American Journal of Clinical Nutrition*, 103(Suppl), 616S–621S.

Lau, C., & Hurst, N. (1999). "Oral feeding in infants." *Current Problems in Pediatrics*, 29(4), 105–124.

Lau, C., Hurst, N. M., Smith, E. O., & Schanler, R. J. (2007). "Ethnic/racial diversity, maternal stress, lactation and very low birthweight infants." *Journal of Perinatology*, 27(7), 399–408.

Lau, C., Alagugurusamy, R., Schanler, R. J., Smith, E. O., & Shulman, R. J. (2000). "Characterization of the developmental stages of sucking in preterm infants during bottle feeding." *Acta Paediatrica*, 89(7), 846–852.

Lee, J., Kim, H. S., Jung, Y. H., Choi, K. Y., Shin, S. H., Kim, E. K., & Choi, J. H. (2015). "Oropharyngeal colostrum administration in extremely premature infants: an RCT." *Pediatrics*, 135(2), e357–366.

Levy, D. M. (1928). "Finger sucking and accessory movements in early infancy." *American Journal of Psychiatry*, 84(6), 881–918.

Mason, S. J., Harris, G., & Blissett, J. (2005). "Tube feeding in infancy: implications for the development of normal eating and drinking skills." *Dysphagia*, 20(1), 46–61.

Mathai, S., Natrajan, N., & Rajalakshmi, N. R. (2006). "A comparative study of non pharmacological methods to reduce pain in neonates." *Indian Pediatrics*, 43(12), 1070–1075.

Mathew, O. P., Clark, M. L., & Pronske, M. H. (1985). "Apnea, bradycardia, and cyanosis during oral feeding in term neonates." *Journal of Pediatrics*, 106(5), 857.

McGowan, J. S., Marsh, R. R., Fowler, S. M., Levy, S. E., & Stallings, V. A. (1991). "Developmental patterns of normal nutritive sucking in infants." *Developmental Medicine and Child Neurology*, 33(10), 891–897.

Melnyk, B. M., Crean, H. F., Feinstein, N. F., & Fairbanks, E. (2008). "Maternal anxiety and depression after a premature infant's discharge from the neonatal intensive care unit: explanatory effects of the creating opportunities for parent empowerment program." *Nursing Research*, 57(6), 383–394.

Meltzoff, A. N., & Moore, M. K. (1977). "Imitation of facial and manual gestures by human neonates." *Science*, 198(4312), 75–78.

Meltzoff, A. N., & Moore, M. K. (1983). "Newborn infants imitate adult facial gestures." *Child Development*, 54(3), 702–709.

Meltzoff, A. N., & Moore, M. K. (1994). "Imitation, memory, and the representation of persons." *Infant Behavior and Development*, 17(1), 83–99.

Meltzoff, A. N., & Moore, M. K. (1997). "Explaining facial imitation: a theoretical model." *Early Development and Parenting*, 6(3–4), 179–192.

Mennella, J. A. (2007). "The chemical senses and the development of flavor preferences in humans." In: T. W. Hale & P. E. Hartmann (eds.), *Hale & Hartmann's Textbook of Human Lactation*. Amarillo, TX: Hale Publishing. pp. 403–414.

Merleau-Ponty, M. (1963). *The Structure of Behavior*. (A. L. Fisher, transl.) Boston, MA: Beacon Press. (Original work published 1942).

Merleau-Ponty, M. (1964). *Signs*. (R. C. McCleary, transl.) Evanston, IL: Northwestern University Press. (Original work published 1960).

Merleau-Ponty, M. (1968). *The Visible and the Invisible*. (A. Lingis, transl.) Evanston, IL: Northwestern University Press. (Original work published 1964).

Merleau-Ponty, M. (2010). *Child Psychology and Pedagogy: The Sorbonne Lectures 1949–1952*. (T. Welsh, transl.) Evanston, IL: Northwestern University Press. (Original work published 2001).

Miles, M. S., Funk, S. G., & Carlson, J. (1993). "Parental stressor scale: neonatal intensive care unit." *Nursing Research*, 42(3), 148–152.

Miller, J. L., Sonies, B. C., & Macedonia, C. (2003). "Emergence of oropharyngeal, laryngeal and swallowing activity in the developing fetal upper aerodigestive tract: an ultrasound evaluation." *Early Human Development*, 71(1), 61–87.

Miller, M. J., & DiFiore, J. M. (1995). "A comparison of swallowing during apnea and periodic breathing in premature infants." *Pediatric Research*, 37(6), 796–799.

Monteagudo, B., & León-Muiños, E. (2010). "Neonatal sucking blisters." *Indian Pediatrics*, 47(9), 794.

Myowa-Yamakoshi, M., & Takeshita, H. (2006). "Do human fetuses anticipate self-oriented actions? A study by four-dimensional (4D) ultrasonography." *Infancy*, 10(3), 289–301.

Nagy, E., Kompagne, H., Orvos, H., & Pal, A. (2007). "Gender related differences in neonatal imitation." *Infant and Child Development*, 16(3), 267–276.

Nagy, E., Kompagne, H., Orvos, H., Pal, A., Molnar, P., Janszky, I., & Bardos, G. (2005). "Index finger movement imitation by human neonates: motivation, learning, and left-hand preference." *Pediatric Research*, 58(4), 749–753.

Piaget, J. (1950). *The Psychology of Intelligence*. San Diego, CA: Harcourt Brace Jovanovich.

Pineda, R., Guth, R., Herring, A., Reynolds, L., Oberle, S., & Smith, J. (2017). "Enhancing sensory experiences for very preterm infants in the NICU: an integrative review." *Journal of Perinatology*, 37(4), 323–332.

Pinelli, J., & Symington, A. (2005). "Non-nutritive sucking for promoting physiologic stability and nutrition in preterm infants." *Cochrane Database of Systematic Reviews*, 4, CD001071

Piontelli, A. (2010). *Development of Normal Fetal Movements: The First 25 Weeks of Gestation*. Milan: Springer-Verlag.

Rattaz, C., Goubet, N., & Bullinger, A. (2005). "The calming effect of a familiar odor on full-term newborns." *Journal of Developmental and Behavioral Pediatrics*, 26(2), 86–92.

Reissland, N. (1988). "Neonatal imitation in the first hour of life: observation in rural Nepal." *Developmental Psychology*, 24(4), 464–469.

Reissland, N., Francis, B., Aydin, E., Mason, J., & Schaal, B. (2014). "The development of anticipation in the fetus: a longitudinal account of human fetal mouth movements in reaction to and anticipation of touch." *Developmental Psychobiology*, 56(5), 955–963.

Righard, L., & Blade, M. O. (1994) "Effect of delivery routines on success of first breast-feed." *Lancet*, 336(8723), 1105–1107.

Rochat, P. (1993). "Hand-mouth coordination in the newborn: morphology, determinants, and early development of a basic act." In: G. J. P. Savelsbergh (ed.), *The Development of Coordination in Infancy*. Amsterdam: North-Holland/Elsevier. pp. 265–288.

Rochat, P. (2003). "Five levels of self-awareness as they unfold early in life." *Consciousness and Cognition*, 12(4), 717–731.

Rochat, P., & Hespos, S. J. (1997). "Differential rooting response by neonates: evidence for an early sense of self." *Early Development and Parenting*, 6(3–4), 105–112.

Rochat, P., Blass, M., & Hoffmeyer, L. B. (1988). "Oropharyngeal control of hand-mouth coordination in newborn infants." *Developmental Psychology*, 24(4), 459–463.

Romano, C. (2015). *At the Heart of Reason*. (M. B. Smith, C. Romano, transl.) Evanston, IL: Northwestern University Press. (Original work published 2010).

Rosen, C. L., Glaze, D. G., & Frost, J. D. Jr. (1984). "Hypoxemia associated with feeding in the preterm infant and full-term neonate." *American Journal of Diseases of Children*, 138 (7), 623–628.

Rovee, C. K., & Levin, G. R. (1966). "Oral 'pacification' and arousal in the human newborn." *Journal of Experimental Child Psychology*, 3(1), 1–17.

Sann, C., & Streri, A. (2007). "Perception of object shape and texture in human new-borns: evidence from cross-modal transfer tasks." *Developmental Science*, 10(3), 399–410.

Sartre, J.-P. (1956). *Being and Nothingness: A Phenomenological Essay on Ontology*. (H. E. Barnes, transl.) New York, NY: Philosophical Library. (Original work published 1943).

Sartre, J.-P. (1991). *The Transcendence of the Ego: An Existentialist Theory of Consciousness*. (F. Williams, R. Kirkpatrick, transl.) New York, NY: Hill & Wang. (Original work published 1937).

Schaal, B., Marlier, L., & Soussignan, R. (1998). "Olfactory function in the human fetus: evidence from selective neonatal responsiveness to the odor of amniotic fluid." *Behavioral Neuroscience*, 112(6), 1438–1449.

Schanler, R. J., Shulman, R. J., Lau, C., Smith, E. O., & Heitkemper, M. M. (1999). "Feeding strategies for premature infants: randomized trial of gastrointestinal priming and tube-feeding method." *Pediatrics*, 103(2), 434–439.

Schloim, N., Vereijken, C. M., Blundell, P., & Hetherington, M. M. (2016). "Looking for cues – infant communication of hunger and satiation during milk feeding." *Appetite*, 108, 74–82.

Schoenfeld, M. A., Neuer, G., Tempelmann, C., Schüssler, K., Noesselt, T., Hopf, J. M., & Heinze, H. J. (2004). "Functional magnetic resonance tomography correlates of taste perception in the human primary taste cortex." *Neuroscience*, 127(2), 347–353.

Simms, E. (2008). *The Child in the World: Embodiment, Time, and Language in Early Childhood*. Detroit, MI: Wayne State University Press.

Simpson, E. A., Murray, L., Paukner, A., & Ferrari, P. F. (2014). "The mirror neuron system as revealed through neonatal imitation: presence from birth, predictive power and evidence of plasticity." *Philosophical Transactions of the Royal Society B: Biological Sciences*, 369(1644), 20130289.

Slater, A., Brown, E., & Badenoch, M. (1997). "Intermodal perception at birth: newborn infants' memory for arbitrary auditory–visual pairings." *Early Development and Parenting*, 6(3–4), 99–104.

Stern, D. N. (1985). *The Interpersonal World of the Infant: A View from Psychoanalysis and Developmental Psychology*. New York, NY: Basic Books.

Streri, A., de Hevia, M. D., Izard, V., & Coubart, A. (2013). "What do we know about neonatal cognition." *Behavioral Sciences*, 3(1), 154–169.

Thakkar, P., Arora, K., Goyal, K., Das, R. R., Javadekar, B., Aiyer, S., & Panigrahi, S. K. (2016). "To evaluate and compare the efficacy of combined sucrose and non-nutritive sucking for analgesia in newborns undergoing minor painful procedure: a randomized controlled trial." *Journal of Perinatology*, 36(1), 67–70.

Trevarthen, C., & Aitken, C. (2003). "Regulation of brain development and age-related changes in infants' motives: the developmental function of regressive periods." In: M. Heimann (ed.), *Regression Periods in Human Infancy*. Mahwah, NJ: Erlbaum. pp. 107–184.

Unruh, A. M. (1992). "Voices from the past: ancient views of pain in childhood." *Clinical Journal of Pain*, 8(3), 247–254.

Van Manen, M. A. (2012). "Technics of touch in the neonatal intensive care." *Medical Humanities*, 38(2), 91–96. Varendi, H., & Porter, R. H. (2001). "Breast odour as the only maternal stimulus elicits crawling towards the odour source." *Acta Paediatrica*, 90(4), 372–375.

Varendi, H., Porter, R. H., & Winberg J. (1994). "Does the newborn baby find the nipple by smell?" *Lancet*, 344(8928), 989–990.

Varendi, H., Porter, R. H., & Winberg, J. (1996). "Attractiveness of amniotic fluid odor: evidence of prenatal olfactory learning?" *Acta Paediatrica*, 85(10), 1223–1227.

Varendi, H., Christensson, K., Porter, R. H., & Winberg, J. (1998). "Soothing effect of amniotic fluid smell in newborn infants." *Early Human Development*, 51(1), 47–55.

Velmans, M., & Schneider, S. (eds.). (2007). *The Blackwell Companion to Consciousness*. Malden, MA: Wiley-Blackwell.

Walker, H. K. (1990). "The suck, snout, palmomental, and grasp reflexes." In: H. K. Walker, W. D. Hall & J. W. Hurst (eds.), *Clinical Methods: The History, Physical, and Laboratory Examinations*. Boston, MA: Butterworths. pp. 363–364.

Waterland, R. A., Berkowitz, R. I., Stunkard, A. J., & Stallings, V. A. (1998). "Calibrated orifice nipples for measurement of infant nutritive sucking." *Journal of Pediatrics*, 132(3 Pt 1), 523–526.

Widström, A.-M., Ransjö-Arvidson, A.-B., Christensson, K., Matthiesen, A.-S., Winberg, J., & Uvnäs-Moberg, K. (1987). "Gastric suction in the newborn infants: effects on circulation and developing feeding behaviours." *Acta Paediatrica Scandinavica*, 76(4), 566–572.

Wolff, P. H. (1968). "The serial organization of sucking in the young infant." *Pediatrics*, 42 (6), 943–956.

Woolridge, M. W. (1986). "The 'anatomy' of infant sucking." *Midwifery*, 2(4), 164–171.

Yan, F., Dai, S. Y., Akther, N., Kuno, A., Yanagihara, T., & Hata, T. (2006). "Four-dimensional sonographic assessment of fetal facial expression early in the third trimester." *International Journal of Gynecology and Obstetrics*, 94(2), 108–113.

Zahavi, D. (2005). *Subjectivity and Selfhood: Investigating the First-Person Perspective*. Cambridge, MA: MIT Press.

Zanardo, V., & Straface, G. (2015). "The higher temperature in the areola supports the natural progression of the birth to breastfeeding continuum." *PLoS ONE*, 10(3), e0118774.

8

BRINGING PHENOMENOLOGY TO PRACTICE

In this book, I have explored the experiential life of the newborn in the transition from womb to world, with particular consideration for newborns requiring medical care. While it might be tempting to attempt to summarize this text with a set of generalizations and conceptual outcomes, that is not the purpose of phenomenological inquiry. Instead, phenomenology aims to raise and deepen questions, cultivate sensitivities, promote thoughtfulness, and present insights of the world as experienced. By way of this questioning, I have aimed to address and speak to the professional and ethical practice of caring for newborns.

As part of their practice, physicians, nurses, and other hospital staff commonly make observations that reflect a particular understanding of the condition of their patients in the NICU. For example, a doctor, a nurse, or other health professional may say that a certain newborn appears 'agitated,' 'unsettled,' or 'in pain.' While I have suggested that it is important to reflect on the taken-for-granted understandings we have of the life of newborns, and in particular of their experiencing of the world, I want to be clear that for ethical practice, a practitioner's experiencing and expressing concern for the wellbeing that is unique to their patient is paramount. Emotive and diagnostic pronouncements are stirred not only by clinical acumen, but also by a fundamental ethical responsiveness and interest in the wellbeing of the patients for whom we care. Such discourse needs to speak to and reflect the ethics of our practice.

We might ask, what is meant by agitation? Is it what we seem to observe in behavior? Or is it what we think the child experiences? Can agitation in itself not be painful? At what point does pain cause agitation? Do we appreciate the possible meanings of being unsettled for a child? Do we grasp the meaning of disorganized behavior, or what we describe when we diagnose a baby as delirious? It is ethically imperative that as practitioners we ask, consider, and wonder what we should do when we say that a newborn is agitated, unsettled, or quite simply in pain—even if we can only incompletely answer such questions. This does not mean that a doctor, nurse, or other caring professional looks at his or her patient with intellectual, objectifying curiosity. But rather, a caregiver sees a patient as having the possibility for a subjective existence very much like his or her own, yet also possibly different from his or her own. Such understanding reflects a constative questioning as an experiential awareness of the possible meaningfulness of the lived experiences of newborns, and also an inquiring wondering based on available research about the developmental capacities of newborns. These empathic gestures ultimately bear on clinical practice.

Pathic Awareness

Much has been written on the complicated subjects of empathy and sympathy from a phenomenological perspective. In the classic text *The Nature of Sympathy*, Max Scheler (1954) offers descriptions of shared or co-feelings: feeling with another (*Miteinanderfühlen*), vicarious feeling (*Nachfühlen*), fellow feeling (*Mitgefühl*), psychic contagion (*Gefühlansteckung*), and identification (*Einsfühlung*). Scheler posits that all of these experiences of feeling are primordial in their lived throughness such that we become conscious of them only after the fact (only after we find ourselves stirred, concerned, upset, joyous, and so forth). We could say that experiences of others that touch our very being reflect a fundamental being-in-the-world with others. Whether we are drawn to others, inclined to participate in the lives of others, or affected by the conditions of others, we live in a social world whereby we may have a fundamental experiential awareness of others.

In her text *On the Problem of Empathy*, Edith Stein (1989) points out that there remains a certain inaccessibility to the subjectivity of another person. She writes about empathy as an "experience of foreign consciousness ... irrespective of the kind of experiencing subject or of the subject whose consciousness is experienced" (p. 11). So, while empathy is "primordial as present experience" (meaning our subjectivity of an other is given in an immediate way free of reflection, deliberation, or questioning as to what that other may be feeling), it is "non-primordial in its content" (meaning the actual subjectivity of an other is not given to us in the same way as it is given to the other; we do not confuse an other's experiencing the world as our own) (p. 10).

When a child cries we may experience the timbre of voice, the expression of face, bodily gestures, and so forth. Still, the child's actual subjective experience of the world (whether it is pain, agitation, or so forth) is not directly available to us. Empathically, we find ourselves feeling alongside an other—yet such awareness does not necessarily eclipse the possibility that this other may experience the world differently. As a nurse, doctor, social worker, or parent, our sensibility and understanding never fully coincides with a newborn. Instead, we have an experiential awareness of bodily gestures and circumstances: "empathy has as its field the sensuous, meaningful experiences of the other's expressions and gestures ... [and lets me] understand the Other's lived body, [thereby] rendering his meanings into my own lived life" (Haney, 1994, p. 59). The "empathic grasp of the other's physically presented meanings is an everyday experience ... which provides the guiding clue" of the other as a psycho-physical, experiencing being, which in turn serves to "open up the moral dimension of empathy" (p. 59).

Although experiential awareness is present in our day-to-day social life, it demands a particular attitude. As healthcare professionals, we may not have empathic experiences if we are focused elsewhere: engaged in a clinical examination, completing a clinical procedure, or making a medical diagnosis. In other words, it is neither unusual nor necessarily amiss for a practitioner to place in abeyance the subjectivity of their patient to focus on their patient as a body. For example, when an infant becomes hypotensive, it is necessary for the practitioner to consider the blood volume status; the filling, functioning, and rhythm of the heart; and, the vascular resistance (i.e., to perceive the newborn more as 'a circulation' than 'a child').

As healthcare professionals, we do not always dwell in attitudes that accommodate an experiential awareness of the possible experiential world of the newborn. Only the empathizing individual is aware that the other to whom he or she relates "has feelings, or is a subject of feelings" (Zahavi, 2001, p. 153). Such understanding is only revealed in an existence that accommodates an "act of a feeling" (Buytendijk, 1987, p. 122). And so, we need to remember that empathy, while being a fundamental experience alongside an other, does not necessarily always occur in our activities with an other. Instead, in the intensive care world of the NICU, it may very well be that we only gain experiential awareness when we look at our patients as newborns, when we are stirred by their subjectivity.

Constative Questioning

A constative questioning aims at understanding the possible subjective experiences of others, recognizing that such understanding necessarily comes from our own personal understanding of the world—and therefore is necessarily exploratory, tentative, and wondering, based on available evidence. Recall that constative reflection is the attempt at phenomenal truth by exploring the meaningfulness of an experience that is based on established empirical evidence.

While we cannot precisely know how a newborn's experiencing of the world resembles that of an adult, it is evident that newborn's existence is meaningful. My assumption has been that engaging with the empirical sciences, their results, descriptions, and findings, may provide useful starting points and topics for reflection. Yet as we engage with the empirical sciences, we need to be careful not to lose sight of the intent of phenomenology:

> Time and again it becomes necessary to impress on ourselves the methodological maxims of phenomenology not to flee prematurely from the enigmatic

character of phenomena nor to explain it away by the violent *coup de main* of a wild theory but rather to accentuate the puzzlement. Only in this way does it become palpable and conceptually comprehensible, that is, intelligible and so concrete that the indications for resolving the phenomenon leap out toward us from the enigmatic matter itself.

(Heidegger, 1988, p. 69)

Constative questioning is not necessarily detached, disconnected, or distant. Nor does it fracture experiences of an other as wholly disparate from our own. After all, the newborn develops to be an adult such that residues of childhood must at the very least mark the being of the adult. Constative reflections teach us that we have to be careful with the qualitative language of our inquiries. Constative expressions require a sensitivity toward the living body of the other since this makes correction of empirical scientific interpretations possible. Some gestures of a newborn we can empathize with ease, while others remain more distant, strange, or puzzling.

We cannot approach the experiences of an other from any other perspective than our own—if we assume or claim something else, we are deluding ourselves (Merleau-Ponty, 1964). Even purely behavioristic approaches always involve subjective dimensions of interpretation that are superficially shaded by the use of objectivistic measures.

They [behavioral scientists] forget that we can understand what has been said only from lived experience and from reality that has become conscious … The world is the birth place, the fertile soil, and the nursery of thought rather than the mere expression of pure ideas or of pre-shaped thought.

(Struyker Boudier, 1986, p. 4)

No matter how seemingly objective our research into newborn behavior, emotions, and consciousness might be, it is nevertheless the case that the adult experience of the newborn is the necessary starting point for any constative consideration of the meaningful substrate of the newborn existence. For example, the multiple pain, agitation, and delirium scales presuppose, overlook, or ignore the meaning or actual *whatness* of newborn pain, agitation, or delirium by reducing the meaning of such named phenomena to scales. This procedural problem does not mean that we should do away with empirical assessments of infant wellbeing; but rather, we need to remember that the claimed objectivity of these scales already presuppose an interpretation of infant subjectivity. We need to ask what are the implications of assessing the wellbeing of a newborn by using a language that objectifies experiential meaning?

Bringing Phenomenology to Practice

Phenomenology of practice is the application of phenomenological inquiry to everyday life concerns "to contribute to more thoughtful practice" (van Manen,

2001, p. 458). The topics of the chapters of this text have been carefully chosen for their significance to the everyday world of newborns requiring medical care. In such research, we need to consider, what 'womb' we are providing to infants born prematurely? We need to ask, what is expressed in the cry of the child? How is eye contact given to the newborn? What may an infant's behavior tell us about their experiential world, even if such behavior appears disorganized to an observer's eyes? These inquiries aim to increase our understanding of the experiential life of the newborn.

For a phenomenology of practice, the intent is not to reduce, objectify, or totalize descriptions of lived experiences; but rather, to gain insight into the meaningfulness of possible human experiences. Indeed, in our professional practice we recognize that our patients and families are all unique, with varied life experiences, predicaments, core values, and so forth. The nurse, doctor, social worker, or other health professional needs to be sensitive to the variety of ways that patient-families may experience their worlds (van Manen, 2014). In other words, practitioners need to ask the simple phenomenological questions in their day-to-day work lives of interacting with their patients, what might this experience be like for them?

Phenomenology can benefit from the discoveries of researchers working with other inquiry paradigms, such as the quantitative, experimental, theoretical, qualitative, and ethical inquiry models. Empirical findings can offer challenges to phenomenological and ontological paradigms, offering new possibilities for exploring lived experiences. Phenomenological method should not be conceptualized as a rigid set of philosophical strategies or techniques. Instead, interpretive methods need to be sensitive to the nuances of particular situations and phenomena. In this text, I have made use of various empirical research findings to try to gain access to the experiential world of the newborn. The hope is that the insights gathered in this text will sponsor conversations between NICU healthcare professionals and families, and that they will support an orientation of care toward the experiential world of the newborn. A phenomenology of practice for the newborn speaks to the ethics of our practice—an openness and appreciation for the meaningfulness of the world of the newborn. If the questioning nature of inquiry is properly acknowledged and appreciated, it can serve as an awakening to the similar-but-different modes of being of the newborn, on the basis of which the meaningfulness of the newborn's world can be attentively explored.

References

Buytendijk, F. J. J. (1987). "The phenomenological approach to the problem of feelings and emotions." In: J. J. Kockelmans (ed.), *Phenomenological Psychology: The Dutch School*. Dordrecht: Martinus Nijhoff Publishers. pp. 119–132.

Haney, K. (1994). "Empathy and ethics." *Southwest Philosophy Review*, 10(1), 57–65.

Heidegger, M. (1988). *The Basic Problems of Phenomenology*. (A. Hofstadter, transl.) Bloomington, IN: Indiana University Press. (Original work published 1975).

Merleau-Ponty, M. (1964). *Sense and Non-Sense*. (H. L. Dreyfus, P. A. Dreyfus, transl.) Evanston, IL: Northwestern University Press. (Original work published 1948).

Scheler, M. (1954). *The Nature of Sympathy*. (P. Heath, transl.) London: Routledge & Kegan Paul. (Original work published 1913).

Stein, E. (1989). *On the Problem of Empathy*. (W. Stein, transl.) Washington, DC: ICS Publications. (Original work published 1917).

Struyker Boudier, C. E. M. (1986). "Merleau-Ponty and Buytendijk: report of a relationship." (R. Rojcewicz, transl.) In: S. Strasser (ed.), *Clefts in the World and Other Essays on Levinas, Merleau-Ponty, and Buytendijk*. Pittsburgh, PA: The Simon Silverman Phenomenology Center Duquesne University. pp. 1–27.

Van Manen, M. (2001). "Professional practice and 'doing phenomenology.'" In: S. Kay Toombs (ed.), *Handbook of Phenomenology and Medicine (Philosophy and Medicine Series)*. Dordrecht: Kluwer Press. pp. 457–474.

Van Manen, M. (2014). *Phenomenology of Practice: Meaning-Giving Methods in Phenomenological Research and Writing*. Walnut Creek, CA: Left Coast Press.

Zahavi, D. (2001). "Beyond empathy: phenomenological approaches to intersubjectivity." *Journal of Consciousness Studies*, 8(5–7), 151–167.

REFERENCES

Abdallah, B., Badr, L. K., & Hawwari, M. (2013). "The efficacy of massage on short and long term outcomes in preterm infants." *Infant Behavior and Development*, 36(4), 662–669.

Achiron, R., Ben Arie, A., Gabbay, U., Mashiach, S., Rotstein, Z., & Lipitz, S. (1997). "Development of the fetal tongue between 14 and 26 weeks of gestation: in utero ultrasonographic measurements." *Ultrasound in Obstetrics & Gynecology*, 9(1), 39–41.

Adamis, D., Treloar, A., Martin, F. C., & Macdonald, A. J. D. (2016). "A brief review of the history of delirium as a mental disorder." *History of Psychiatry*, 18(4), 459–469.

Adolph, K. E., & Berger, S. E. (2015). "Physical and motor development." In: M. H. Bornstein & M. E. Lamb (eds.), *Developmental Science: An Advanced Textbook, 7th edition*. New York, NY: Psychology Press. pp. 261–333.

Als, H. (1977). "The newborn communicates." *Journal of Communication*, 27(2), 66–73.

Als, H. (1982). "Toward a synactive theory of development: promise for the assessment of infant individuality." *Infant Mental Health Journal*, 3(4), 229–243.

Als, H., & Brazelton, T. B. (1981). "A new model of assessing the behavioral organization in preterm and fullterm infants." *Journal of the American Academy of Child Psychiatry*, 20 (2), 239–263.

Amaizu, N., Shulman, R., Schanler, R., & Lau, C. (2008). "Maturation of oral feeding skills in preterm infants." *Acta Paediatrica*, 97(1), 61–67.

American Psychiatric Association. (1981). *Diagnostic and Statistical Manual of Mental Disorders, 3rd Edition*. Washington, DC: American Psychiatric Association.

American Psychiatric Association. (1987). *Diagnostic and Statistical Manual of Mental Disorders: DSM-IIIR*. Washington, DC: American Psychiatric Association.

American Psychiatric Association. (1994). *Diagnostic and Statistical Manual of Mental Disorders: DSM-IV*. Washington, DC: American Psychiatric Association.

American Psychiatric Association. (2000). *Diagnostic and Statistical Manual of Mental Disorders: DSM-IV-TR*. Washington, DC: American Psychiatric Association.

American Psychiatric Association. (2013). *Diagnostic and Statistical Manual of Mental Disorders: DSM-5*. Arlington, VA: American Psychiatric Association.

Amiel-Tison, C., & Grenier, A. (1980). *Evaluation Neurologique du Nouveau-né et du Nourrisson*. Paris: Masson.

Anand, K. J. S., & Hall, R. W. (2008). "Love, pain, and intensive care." *Pediatrics*, 121(4), 825–827.

Anand, K. J., & Hickey, P. R. (1987). "Pain and its effects in the human neonate and fetus." *New England Journal of Medicine*, 317(21), 1321–1329.

Anand, K. J., Sippel, W. G., & Aynsley-Green, A. (1987). "Randomised trial of fentanyl anasethesia in preterm babies undergoing surgery: effects on the stress response." *Lancet*, 329(8527), 243–248.

Anand, K. J., Brown, M. J., Bloom, S. R., & Aynsley-Green, A. (1985). "Studies on the hormonal regulation of fuel metabolism in the human newborn infant undergoing anaesthesia and surgery." *Hormone Research*, 22(1–2), 115–128.

Anand, K. J., Barton, B. A., McIntosh, N., Lagercrantz, H., Pelausa, E., Young, T. E., & Vasa, R. (1999). "Analgesia and sedation in preterm neonates who require ventilator support: results from the NOPAIN trial: neonatal outcome and prolonged analgesia in neonates." *Archives of Pediatrics & Adolescent Medicine*, 153(4), 331–338.

Anand, K. J., Hall, R. W., Desai, N., Shephard, B., Bergqvist, L. L., Young, T. E., Boyle, E. M., Carbajal, R., Bhutani, V. K., Moore, M. B., Kronsberg, S. S., & Barton, B. A.; NEOPAIN Trial Investigators Group. (2004). "Effects of morphine analgesia in ventilated preterm neonates: primary outcomes from the NEOPAIN randomised trial." *Lancet*, 363(9422), 1673–1682.

Andersson, E. M., Hallberg, I. R., Norberg, A., & Edberg, A. K. (2002). "The meaning of acute confusional state from the perspective of elderly patients." *International Journal of Geriatric Psychiatric*, 17(7), 652–663.

Apgar, V. (1953). "A proposal for a new method for evaluation of the newborn infant." *Current Researchers in Anesthesia & Analgesia*, 32(4), 260–267.

Asakura, H. (2004). "Fetal and neonatal thermoregulation." *Journal of Nippon Medical School*, 71(6), 360–370.

Atkinson, J. (1984). "Human visual development over the first six months of life: a review and a hypothesis." *Human Neurobiology*, 3(2), 61–74.

Augustine. (2012). *The City of God*. (W. Babcock, transl.) Hyde Park, NY: New City Press. (Original work published 426 AD).

Azañón, E., Camacho, K., Morales, M., & Longo, M. R. (2017). "The sensitive period for tactile remapping does not include early infancy." *Child Development*, 89(4), 1394–1404. doi:10.1111/cdev.12813

Azarmnejad, E., Sarhangi, F., Javadi, M., & Rejeh, N. (2015). "The effect of mother's voice on arterial blood sampling induced pain in neonates hospitalized in neonate intensive care unit." *Global Journal of Health Science*, 7(6), 198–204.

Bachelard, G. (1994). *The Poetics of Space*. (M. Jolas, transl.) Boston, MA: Beacon Press. (Original work published 1958).

Badiee, Z., Asghari, M., & Mohammadizadeh, M. (2013). "The calming effect of maternal breast milk odor on premature infants." *Pediatrics and Neonatology*, 54(5), 322–325.

Barlow, S. M., Dusick, A., Finan, D. S., Coltart, S., & Biswas, A. (2001). "Mechanically evoked perioral reflexes in premature and term infants." *Brain Research*, 899(1–2), 251–254.

Bartocci, M., Bergqvist, L. L., Lagercrantz, H., & Anand, K. J. (2006). "Pain activates cortical areas in the preterm newborn brain." *PAIN*, 122(1–2), 109–117.

Bartocci, M., Winberg, J., Papendieck, G., Mustica, T., Serra, G., & Lagercrantz, H. (2001). "Cerebral hemodynamic response to unpleasant odors in the preterm newborn measured by near-infrared spectroscopy." *Pediatric Research*, 50(3), 324–330.

Bartocci, M., Winberg, J., Ruggiero, C., Bergqvist, L. L., Serra, G., & Lagercrantz, H. (2000). "Activation of olfactory cortex in newborn infants after odor stimulation: a functional near-infrared spectroscopy study." *Pediatric Research*, 48(1), 18–23.

Batki, A., Baron-Cohen, S., Wheelwright, S., Connellan, J., & Ahluwalia, J. (2000). "Is there an innate gaze module? Evidence from human neonates." *Infant Behavior and Development*, 23(2), 223–229.

Bauer, P. J. (2006). "Constructing a past in infancy: a neuro-developmental account." *Trends in Cognitive Sciences*, 10(4), 175–191.

Bayley, J.; Committee on Fetus and Newborn. (2015). "Skin-to-skin care for preterm infants in the neonatal ICU." *Pediatrics*, 136(3), 596–599.

Baylis, R., Ewald, U., Gradin, M., Hedberg Nyqvist, K., Rubertsson, C., & Thernström Blomqvist, Y. (2014). "First-time events between parents and preterm infants are affected by the designs and routines of neonatal intensive care units." *Acta Paediatrica*, 103 (10), 1045–1052.

Beijers, R., Buitelaar, J. K., & de Weerth, C. (2014). "Mechanisms underlying the effects of prenatal psychosocial stress on child outcomes: beyond the HPA axis." *European Child & Adolescent Psychiatry*, 23(10), 943–956.

Birnholz, J. C., & Benacerraf, B. R. (1983). "The development of human fetal hearing." *Science*, 222(4623), 516–518.

Blass, E. M., Fillion, T. J., Rochat, P., Hoffmeyer, L. B., & Metzger, M. A. (1989). "Sensorimotor and motivational determinants of hand-mouth coordination in 1–3-day-old human infants." *Developmental Psychology*, 25(6), 963–975.

Boere, I., Roest, A. A., Wallace, E., Ten Harkel, A. D., Haak, M. C., Morley, C. J., Hooper, S. B., & te Pas, A. B. (2015). "Umbilical blood flow patterns directly after birth before delayed cord clamping." *Archives of Disease in Childhood. Fetal and Neonatal Edition*, 100(2), F121–125.

Borenstein-Levin, L., Synnes, A., Grunau, R. E., Miller, S. P., Yoon, E. W., & Shah, P. S.; Canadian Neonatal Network Investigators. (2017). "Narcotics and sedative use in preterm neonates." *Journal of Pediatrics*, 180, 92–98.

Branco, A., Behlau, M., & Rehder, M. A. (2005). "The neonatal cry after caesarean section and vaginal delivery during the first minutes of life." *International Journal of Pediatric Otorhinolaryngology*, 69(5), 681–689.

Brazelton, T. B. (1985). "Application of cry research to clinical perspectives." In: B. M. Lester & C. F. Zachariah Boukydis (eds.), *Infant Crying: Theoretical and Research Perspectives*. New York, NY: Plenum Press. pp. 325–340.

Broome, M. E., & Tanzillo, H. (1990). "Differentiating between pain and agitation in premature neonates." *Journal of Perinatal Neonatal Nursing*, 4(1), 53–62.

Brummelte, S., Grunau, R. E., Chau, V., Poskitt, K. J., Brant, R., Vinall, J., Gover, A., Synnes, A. R., & Miller, S. P. (2012). "Procedural pain and brain development in premature newborns." *Annals of Neurology*, 71(3), 385–396.

Burra, N., Hervais-Adelman, A., Kerzel, D., Tamietto, M., de Gelder, B., & Pegna, A. J. (2013). "Amygdala activation for eye contact despite complete cortical blindness." *The Journal of Neuroscience*, 33(25), 10483–10489.

Busnel, M. (1979). "Intravaginal measurements of the level and acoustic distortion of maternal noises." *Electrodiagnostic-Therapie*, 16(3), 142.

Butterworth, G., & Hopkins, B. (1988). "Hand-mouth coordination in the new-born baby." *British Journal of Developmental Psychology*, 6(4), 303–314.

Buytendijk, F. J. J. (1953). "Experienced freedom and moral freedom in the child's consciousness." *Educational Theory*, 3(1), 1–13.

Buytendijk, F. J. J. (1974). *Prolegomena to an Anthropological Physiology*. Pittsburgh, PA: Duquesne University Press. (Original work published 1965).

Buytendijk, F. J. J. (1987). "The phenomenological approach to the problem of feelings and emotions." In: J. J. Kockelmans (ed.), *Phenomenological Psychology: The Dutch School*. Dordrecht: Martinus Nijhoff Publishers. pp. 119–132.

Buytendijk, F. J. J. (1988). "The first smile of the child." *Phenomenology + Pedagogy*, 6(1), 15–24.

Carbajal, R., Chauvet, X., Couderc, S., & Olivier-Martin, M. (1999). "Randomised trial of analgesic effects of sucrose, glucose, and pacifiers in term neonates." *British Medical Journal*, 319(7222), 1393–1397.

Carbajal, R., Rousset, A., Danan, C., Coquery, S., Nolent, P., Ducrocq, S., Saizou, C., Lapillonne, A., Granier, M., Durand, P., Lenclen, R., Coursol, A., Hubert, P., de Saint Blanquat, L., Boëlle, P. Y., Annequin, D., Cimerman, P., Anand, K. J., & Bréart, G. (2008). "Epidemiology and treatment of painful procedures in neonates in intensive care units." *JAMA*, 300(1), 60–70.

Carbajal, R., Eriksson, M., Courtois, E., Boyle, E., Avila-Alvarez, A., Andersen, R. D., Sarafidis, K., Polkki, T., Matos, C., Lago, P., Papadouri, T., Montalto, S. A., Ilmoja, M. L., Simon, S., Tameliene, R., van Overmeire, B., Berger, A., Dobrzanska, A., Schroth, M., Bergqvist, L., Lagercrantz, H., & Anand, K. J.; EUROPAIN Survey Working Group. (2015). "Sedation and analgesia practices in neonatal intensive care units (EUROPAIN): results from a prospective cohort study." *The Lancet Respiratory Medicine*, 3(10), 796–812.

Carter, B. S., & Brunkhorst, J. (2017). "Neonatal pain management." *Seminars in Perinatology*, 41(2), 111–116.

Casey, E. S. (2000). *Remembering: A Phenomenological Study*. Bloomington, IN: Indiana University Press.

Castiello, U., Becchio, C., Zoia, S., Nelini, C., Sartori, L., Blason, L., D'Ottavio, G., Bulgheroni, M., & Gallese, V. (2010). "Wired to be social: the ontogeny of human interaction." *PLOS One*, 5(10), e13199.

Castral, T. C., Warnock, F., Leite, A. M., Haas, V. J., & Scochi, C. G. (2008). "The effects of skin-to-skin contact during acute pain in preterm newborns." *European Journal of Pain*, 12(4), 464–471.

Cecchini, M., Baroni, E., Di Vito, C., & Lai, C. (2011b). "Smiling in newborns during communicative wake and active sleep." *Infant Behavior & Development*, 34(3), 417–423.

Cecchini, M., Baroni, E., Di Vito, C., Piccolo, F., & Lai, C. (2011a). "Newborn preference for a new face vs. a previously seen communicative or motionless face." *Infant Behavior & Development*, 34(3), 424–433.

Chan, G. J., Valsangkar, B., Kajeepeta, S., Boundy, E. O., & Wall, S. (2016). "What is kangaroo mother care? Systematic review of the literature." *Journal of Global Health*, 6(1), 010701.

Charil, A., Laplante, D. P., Vaillancourt, C., & King, S. (2010). "Prenatal stress and brain development." *Brain Research Reviews*, 65(1), 56–79.

Chau, V., Taylor, M. J., & Miller, S. P. (2013). "Visual function in preterm infants: visualizing the brain to improve prognosis." *Documenta Ophthalmologica*, 127(1), 41–55.

Chen, K. L., Quah-Smith, I., Schmölzer, G. M., Niemtzow, R., & Oei, J. L. (2017). "Acupuncture in the neonatal intensive care unit-using ancient medicine to help today's babies: a review." *Journal of Perinatology*, 37(7), 749–756.

Chen, Y.-C., Lewis, T. L., Shore, D. I., & Maurer, D. (2017). "Early binocular input is critical for development of audiovisual but not visualtactile simultaneity perception." *Current Biology*, 27(4), 583–589.

Christensson, K., Cabrera, T., Christensson, E., Uvnäs-Moberg, K., & Winberg, J. (1995). "Separation distress call in the human neonate in the absence of maternal body contact." *Acta Paediatrica*, 84(5), 468–473.

Clark-Gambelunghe, M. B., & Clark, D. A. (2015). "Sensory development." *Pediatric Clinics of North America*, 62(2), 367–384.

Cooper, R. P., & Aslin, R. N. (1989). "The language environment of the young infant: implications for early perceptual development." *Canadian Journal of Psychology*, 43(2), 247–265.

Crossley, K. J., Allison, B. J., Polglase, G. R., Morley, C. J., Davis, P. G., & Hooper, S. B. (2009). "Dynamic changes in the direction of blood flow through the ductus arteriosus at birth." *The Journal of Physiology*, 587(Pt 19), 4695–4704.

D'Elia, A., Pighetti, M., Moccia, G., & Santangelo, N. (2001). "Spontaneous motor activity in normal fetuses." *Early Human Development*, 65(2), 139–147.

Darwin, C. R. (1989). *The Expression of the Emotions in Man and Animals*. New York, NY: New York University Press. (Original work published 1872).

De Graaf, J., van Lingen, R. A., Valkenburg, A. J., Weisglas-Kuperus, N., Groot Jebbink, L., Wijnberg-Williams, B., Anand, K. J., Tibboel, D., & van Dijk, M. (2013). "Does neonatal morphine use affect neuropsychological outcomes at 8 to 9 years of age?" *PAIN*, 154(3), 449–458.

De Graaf, J., van Lingen, R. A., Simons, S. H., Anand, K. J., Duivenvoorden, H. J., Weisglas-Kuperus, N., Roofthooft, D. W., Groot Jebbink, L. J., Veenstra, R. R., Tibboel, D., & van Dijk, M. (2011). "Long-term effects of routine morphine infusion in mechanically ventilated neonates on children's functioning: five year follow-up of a randomized controlled trial." *PAIN*, 152(6), 1391–1397.

De Vries, J. I., Visser, G. H., & Prechtl, H. F. (1982). "The emergence of fetal behaviour: I. Qualitative aspects." *Early Human Development*, 7(4), 301–322.

De Vries, J. I., Visser, G. H., & Prechtl, H. F. (1985). "The emergence of fetal behaviour. II. Quantitative aspects." *Early Human Development*, 12(2), 99–120.

De Vries, J. I. P., Visser, G. H. A., & Prechtl, H. F. R. (1988). "The emergence of fetal behaviour. III. Individual differences and consistencies." *Early Human Development*, 16(1), 85–103.

De Vries, J. I., Visser, G. H., Mulder, E. J., & Prechtl, H. F. (1987). "Diurnal and other variations in fetal movements and heart rate patterns at 20–22 weeks." *Early Human Development*, 15(6), 333–348.

DeCasper, A. J., & Fifer, W. P. (1980). "Of human bonding: newborns prefer their mothers' voices." *Science*, 208(4448), 1174–1176.

DeCasper, A. J., & Spence, M. J. (1986). "Prenatal maternal speech influences newborn's perception of speech sounds." *Infant Behavior and Development*, 9(2), 133–150.

DeCasper, A. J., Lecanuet, J.-P., Busnel, M.-C., Granier-Deferre, C., & Maugeais, R. (1994). "Fetal reactions to recurrent maternal speech." *Infant Behavior and Development*, 17(2), 159–164.

Descroix, E., Charavel, M., Świątkowski, W., & Graff, C. (2015) "Spontaneous eye-blinking rate from pre-term to six-months." *Cogent Psychology* (serial online), 2(1), 1–14.

DiPietro, J. A., Irizarry, R. A., Costigan, K. A., & Gurewitsch, E. D. (2004). "The psychophysiology of the maternal-fetal relationship." *Psychophysiology*, 41(4), 510–520.

Donaldson, M. (1993). *Human Minds: An Exploration*. London: Allen Lane, The Penguin Press.

Dondi, M., Messinger, D., Colle, M., Tabasso, A., Simion, F., Dalla Barba, B., & Fogel, A. (2007). "A new perspective in neonatal smiling: differences between the judgments of expert coders and naive observers." *Infancy*, 12(3), 235–255.

Draganova, R., Eswaran, H., Murphy, P., Lowery, C., & Preissl, H. (2007). "Serial magnetoencephalographic study of fetal newborn auditory discriminative evoked responses." *Early Human Development*, 83(3), 199–207.

Dubowitz, L. M., Mushin, J., De Vries, L., & Arden, G. B. (1986). "Visual function in the newborn infant: is it cortically mediated?" *Lancet*, 1(8490), 1139–1141.

Dukhovny, D., Pursley, D. M., Kirpalani, H. M., Horbar, J. H., & Zupancic, J. A. (2016). "Evidence, quality, and waste: solving the value equation in neonatology." *Pediatrics*, 137(3), e20150312.

Duppils, G. S., & Wikblad, K. (2007). "Patients' experiences of being delirious." *Journal of Clinical Nursing*, 16(5), 810–818.

Durier, V., Henry, S., Martin, E., Dollion, N., Hausberger, M., & Sizun, J. (2015). "Unexpected behavioural consequences of preterm newborns' clothing." *Scientific Reports*, 5, 9177.

Dutton, G. N. (2013). "The spectrum of cerebral visual impairment as a sequel to premature birth: an overview." *Documenta Ophthalmologica*, 127(1), 69–78.

Eichenwald, E. C., Blackwell, M., Lloyd, J. S., Tran, T., Wilker, R. E., & Richardson, D. K. (2001). "Inter-neonatal intensive care unit variation in discharge timing: influence of apnea and feeding management." *Pediatrics*, 108(4), 928–933.

Ekman, P., Davidson, R. J., & Friesen, W. V. (1990). "The Duchenne smile: emotional expression and brain physiology II." *Journal of Personality and Social Psychology*, 58(2), 342–353.

European Delirium Association & American Delirium Society. (2014). "The DSM-5 criteria, level of arousal and delirium diagnosis: inclusiveness is safer." *BMC Medicine*, 12, 141.

Fabrizi, L., Slater, R., Worley, A., Meek, J., Boyd, S., Olhede, S., & Fitzgerald, M. (2011). "A shift in sensory processing that enables the developing human brain to discriminate touch from pain." *Current Biology*, 21(18), 1552–1558.

Fagerberg, I., & Jönhagen, M. E. (2002). "Temporary confusion: a fearful experience." *Journal of Psychiatric and Mental Health Nursing*, 9(3), 339–346.

Fantz, R. (1961). "The origin of form perception." *Scientific American*, 204, 66–72.

Farroni, T., Menon, E., & Johnson, M. H. (2006). "Factors influencing newborns' preference for faces with eye contact." *Journal of Experimental Child Psychology*, 95(4), 298–308.

Farroni, T., Gergely, C., Simion, F., & Johnson, M. H. (2002). "Eye contact detection in humans from birth." *Proceedings of the National Academy of Sciences*, 99(14), 9603–9605.

Field, T. M., Woodson, R., Greenberg, R., & Cohen, D. (1982). "Discrimination and imitation of facial expressions by neonates." *Science*, 218(4568), 179–181.

Field, T. M., Woodson, R., Cohen, D., Greenberg, R., Garcia, R., & Collins, K. (1983). "Discrimination and imitation of facial expressions by term and preterm neonates." *Infant Behavior and Development*, 6(4), 485–489.

Fifer, W. P., & Moon, C. M. (1995). "The effects of fetal experience with sound." In: J. P. Lecanuet, W. P. Fifer, N. A. Krasnegor, & W. P. Smotherman (eds.), *Fetal Development: A Psychobiological Perspective*. Hillsdale, NJ: Lawrence Erlbaum Associates. pp. 351–366.

Fischer, C., Rybakowski, C., Ferdynus, C., Sagot, P., & Gouyon, J. B. (2012). "A population-based study of meconium aspiration syndrome in neonates born between 37 and 43 weeks of gestation." *International Journal of Pediatrics*, 321545.

Fitzgerald, M. (2015). "What do we really know about newborn infant pain?" *Experimental Physiology*, 100(12), 1451–1457.

Fort, A., & Manfredi, C. (1998). "Acoustic analysis of newborn infant cry signals." *Medical Engineering & Physics*, 20(6), 432–442.

Foster, J. P., Psaila, K., & Patterson, T. (2016). "Non-nutritive sucking for increasing physiologic stability and nutrition in preterm infants." *Cochrane Database of Systematic Reviews*, 10, CD001071.

Gadamer, H.-G. (2004). *Truth and Method*. (J. Weinsheimer, D. G. Marshall, transl.) London: Continuum. (Original work published 1975).

Gallese, V., Fadiga, L., Fogassi, L., & Rizzolatti, G. (1996). "Action recognition in the premotor cortex." *Brain*, 119(Pt 2), 593–609.

Gibbins, S., Stevens, B., McGrath, P. J., Yamada, J., Beyene, J., Breau, L., Camfield, C., Finley, A., Franck, L., Johnston, C., Howlett, A., McKeever, P., O'Brien, K., & Ohlsson, A. (2008). "Comparison of pain responses in infants of different gestational ages." *Neonatology*, 93(1), 10–18.

Giganti, F., Ficca, G., Cioni, G., & Salzarulo, P. (2006). "Spontaneous awakenings in preterm and term infants assessed throughout 24-h video-recordings." *Early Human Development*, 82(7), 435–440.

Gingras, J. L., Mitchell, E. A., & Grattan, K. E. (2005). "Fetal homologue of infant crying." *Archives of Disease in Childhood. Fetal and Neonatal Edition*, 90(5), F415–F418.

Giorgi, A. (1970). *Psychology as a Human Science: A Phenomenologically Based Approach*. New York, NY: Harper & Row.

Giorgi, A. (2009). *The Descriptive Phenomenological Method in Psychology: A Modified Husserlian Approach*. Pittsburgh, PA: Duquesne University Press.

Goberman, A. M., & Robb, M. P. (1999). "Acoustic examination of preterm and full-term infant cries: the long-time average spectrum." *Journal of Speech, Language, and Hearing Research*, 42(4), 850–861.

Goren, C. C., Sarty, M., & Wu, P. Y. K. (1975). "Visual following and pattern discrimination of face-like stimuli by newborn infants." *Pediatrics*, 56(4), 544–549.

Granier-Deferre, C., Bassereau, S., Ribeiro, A., Jacquet, A.-Y., & DeCasper, A. J. (2011). "A melodic contour repeatedly experienced by human near-term fetuses elicits a profound cardiac reaction one month after birth." *PLoS ONE*, 6(2), e17304.

Groves, A., Traube, C., & Silver, G. (2016). "Detection and management of delirium in the neonatal unit: a case series." *Pediatrics*, 137(3), e20153369.

Grover, S., Malhotra, S., Bharadwaj, R., Bn, S., & KumarS. (2009). "Delirium in children and adolescents." *International Journal of Psychiatry in Medicine*, 39(2), 179–187.

Grunau, R. V. E., & Craig, K. D. (1987). "Pain expression in neonates: facial action and cry." *PAIN*, 28(3), 395–410.

Grunau, R. E., Oberlander, T. F., Whitfield, M. F., Fitzgerald, C., & Lee, S. K. (2001). "Demographic and therapeutic determinants of pain reactivity in very low birth weight neonates at 32 weeks' postconceptional age." *Pediatrics*, 107(1), 105–112.

Haney, K. (1994). "Empathy and ethics." *Southwest Philosophy Review*, 10(1), 57–65.

Hatherill, S., & Flisher, A. J. (2010). "Delirium in children and adolescents: a systematic review of the literature." *Journal of Psychosomatic Research*, 68(4), 337–344.

Heidegger, M. (1962). *Being and Time*. (J. Macquarrie, E. Robinson, transl.) New York, NY: Harper & Row. (Original work published 1927).

Heidegger, M. (1988). *The Basic Problems of Phenomenology*. (A. Hofstadter, transl.) Bloomington, IN: Indiana University Press. (Original work published 1975).

Heidegger, M. (1995) *The Fundamental Concepts of Metaphysics: World, Finitude, Solitude*. (W. McNeill, N. Walker, transl.) Bloomington, IN: Indiana University Press. (Original work published 1983).

Heidegger, M. (2012). *Contributions to Philosophy (of the Event)*. (R. Rojcewicz, D. Vallega-Neu, transl.) Bloomington, IN: Indiana University Press. (Original work published 1989).

Henry, M. (2008). *Material Phenomenology*. (S. Davidson, transl.) New York, NY: Fordham University Press. (Original work published 1990).

Henry, M. (2009). *Seeing the Invisible: On Kandinsky*. (S. Davidson, transl.) New York, NY: Continuum. (Original work published 1988).

Hepper, P. G. (1988). "Fetal 'soap' addiction." *Lancet*, 1(8598), 1347–1348.

Hepper, P., Scott, D., & Shahidullah, S. (1993). "Newborn and fetal response to maternal voice." *Journal of Reproductive and Infant Psychology*, 11(3), 147–155.

Hepper, P. G., Shahidullah, S., & White, R. (1991). "Handedness in the human fetuses." *Neuropsychologia*, 29(11), 1107–1111.

Herrington, C. J., & Chiodo, L. M. (2014). "Human touch effectively and safely reduces pain in the newborn intensive care unit." *Pain Management Nursing*, 15(1), 107–115.

Hillman, N. H., Kallapur, S. G., & Jobe, A. H. (2012). "Physiology of transition from intrauterine to extrauterine life." *Clinical Perinatology*, 39(4), 769–783.

Holst, M., Eswaran, H., Lowery, C., Murphy, P., Norton, J., & Preissl, H. (2005). "Development of auditory evoked fields in human fetuses newborns: a longitudinal MEG study." *Clinical Neurophysiology*, 116(8), 1949–1955.

Hooper, S. B., & Harding, R. (2005). "Role of aeration in the physiological adaptation of the lung to air breathing at birth." *Current Respiratory Medicine Reviews*, 1(2), 185–195.

Hooper, S. B., Polglase, G. R., & te Pas, A. B. (2015). "A physiological approach to the timing of umbilical cord clamping at birth." *Archives of Disease in Childhood. Fetal and Neonatal Edition*, 100(4), F355–360.

Horimoto, N., Koyanagi, T., Nagata, S., Nakahara, H., & Nakano, H. (1989). "Concurrence of mouthing movement and rapid eye movement/non-rapid eye movement phases with advance in gestation of the human fetus." *American Journal of Obstetrics & Gynecology*, 161(2), 344–351.

Hummel, P., Puchalski, M., Creech, S. D., & Weiss, M. G. (2008). "Clinical reliability and validity of the N-PASS: neonatal pain, agitation and sedation scale with prolonged pain." *Journal of Perinatology*, 28(1), 55–60.

Humphrey, T. (1970). "Reflex activity in the oral and facial area of the human fetus." In: J. F. Bosma (ed.), *Second Symposium on Oral Sensation and Perception*. Springfield, IL: Charles C. Thomas. pp. 195–233.

Hunter, C. J., Bennet, L., Power, G. G., Roelfsema, V., Blood, A. B., Quaedackers, J. S., George, S., Guan, J., & Gunn, A. J. (2003). "Key neuroprotective role for endogenous adenosine A1 receptor activation during asphyxia in the fetal sheep." *Stroke*, 34(9), 2240–2245.

Husserl, E. (1989). *Ideas Pertaining to a Pure Phenomenology and to a Phenomenological Philosophy. Second Book: General Introduction to a Pure Phenomenology*. (R. Rojcewicz, A. Schuwer, transl.) Dordrecht: Kluwer. (Original work published 1913).

Husserl, E. (1991). *On the Phenomenology of the Consciousness of Internal Time (1893–1917)*. (J. B. Brough, transl.) Dordrecht: Kluwer Academic. (Original work published 1966).

Husserl, E. (2001). *Logical Investigations, Volume 1*. (J. N. Findlay, transl.) Oxon: Routledge. (Original work published 1900/1901).

Ihde, D. (1990). *Technology and the Lifeworld: From Garden to Earth*. Bloomington, IN: Indiana University Press.

Jackson, B. N., Kelly, B. N., McCann, C. M., & Purdy, S. C. (2016). "Predictors of the time to attain full oral feeding in late preterm infants." *Acta Paediatrica*, 105(1), e1–6.

Jackson, I. M. (1943). "Cry of the child in utero." *British Medical Journal*, 2(4312), 266–267.

James, W. (1890). *Principles of Psychology*. New York, NY: Henry Holt and Company.

Jandó, G., Mikó-Baráth, E., Markó, K., Hollódy, K., Török, B., & Kovacs, I. (2012). "Early-onset binocularity in preterm infants reveals experience-dependent visual development in humans." *Proceedings of the National Academy of Sciences*, 109(27), 11049–11052.

Jensen, K. (1932). "Differential reactions to taste and temperature stimuli in newborn infants." *Genetic Psychological Monographs*, 12(5–6), 363–479.

Johnson, M. (2007). *The Meaning of the Body: Aesthetics of Human Understanding*. Chicago, IL: University of Chicago Press.

Johnson, M. H., & Morton, J. (1991). *Biology and Cognitive Development: The Case of Face Recognition*. Oxford: Blackwell.

Johnston, C. C., & Stevens, B. J. (1996). "Experience in a neonatal intensive care unit affects pain response." *Pediatrics*, 98(5), 925–930.

Johnston, C., Barrington, K. J., Taddio, A., Carbajal, R., & Filion, F. (2011). "Pain in Canadian NICUs: have we improved over the past 12 years?" *Clinical Journal of Pain*, 27 (3), 225–232.

Johnston, C., Campbell-Yeo, M., Disher, T., Benoit, B., Fernandes, A., Streiner, D., Inglis, D., & Zee, R. (2017). "Skin-to-skin care for procedural pain in neonates." *Cochrane Database of Systematic Reviews*, 2, CD008435.

Jones, S. (2017). "Can newborn infants imitate?" *Wiley Interdisciplinary Reviews: Cognitive Science*, 8(1–2), e1410.

Kawakami, F., & Yanaihara, T. (2012). "Smiles in the fetal period." *Infant Behavior and Development*, 35(3), 466–471.

Kawakami, K., Takai-Kawakami, K., Kawakami, F., Tomonaga, M., Suzuki, M., & Shimizu, Y. (2008). "Roots of smile: a preterm neonates' study." *Infant Behavior and Development*, 31(3), 518–522.

Kaye, H. (1967). "Infant sucking behavior and its modification." *Advances in Child Development and Behavior*, 3, 1–52.

Kisilevsky, B. S., Hains, S. M., Lee, K., Xie, X., Huang, H., Ye, H. H., Zhang, K., & Wang, Z. (2003). "Effects of experience on fetal voice recognition." *Psychological Science*, 14(3), 220–224.

Kitzmiller, J. L., & Mitchell, W. B. (1942). "Vagitus uterinus." *Western Journal of Surgery, Obstetrics, and Gynecology*, 50, 620–621.

Klaus, M. (1998). "Mother and infant: early emotional ties." *Pediatrics*, 102(sup E1), 1244–1246.

Koenig, J. S., Davies, A. M., & Thach, B. T. (1990). "Coordination of breathing, sucking, and swallowing during bottle feedings in human infants." *Journal of Applied Physiology*, 69(5), 1623–1629.

Krechel, S. W., & Bildner, J. (1995). "CRIES: a new neonatal postoperative pain measurement score. Initial testing of validity and reliability." *Pediatric Anesthesia*, 5(1), 53–61.

Kucukoglu, S., Kurt, S., & Aytekin, A. (2015). "The effect of the facilitated tucking position in reducing vaccination-induced pain in newborns." *Italian Journal of Pediatrics*, 41, 61.

Kucukoglu, S., Aytekin, A., Celebioglu, A., Celebi, A., Caner, I., & Maden, R. (2016). "Effect of white noise in relieving vaccination pain in premature infants." *Pain Management Nursing*, 17(6), 392–400.

Kuperus, G. (2007). "Attunement, deprivation, and drive: Heidegger and animality." In: C. Lotz & C. Painter (eds.), *Phenomenology and the Non-Human Animal: At the Limits of Experience*. Dordrecht: Sage. pp. 13–27.

Kurjak, A., Azumendi, G., Vecek, N., Kupesic, S., Solak, M., Varga, D., & Chervenak, F. (2003). "Fetal hand movements and facial expression in normal pregnancy studied by four-dimensional sonography." *Journal of Perinatal Medicine*, 31(6), 496–508.

Lagercrantz, H. (2014). "The emergence of consciousness: science and ethics." *Seminars of Fetal and Neonatal Medicine*, 19(5), 300–305.

Lagercrantz, H., & Changeux, J.-P. (2009). "The emergence of human consciousness: from fetal to neonatal life." *Pediatric Research*, 65(3), 255–260.

Lagercrantz, H., & Changeux, J. P. (2010). "Basic consciousness of the newborn." *Seminars in Perinatology*, 34(3), 201–206.

Laitinen, H. (1996). "Patients' experience of confusion in the intensive care unit following cardiac surgery." *Intensive and Critical Care Nursing*, 12(2), 79–83.

Lambert, S. R., & Drack, A. V. (1996). "Infantile cataracts." *Survey of Ophthalmology*, 40(6), 427–458.

Lang, P. J. (1994). "The varieties of emotional experience: a meditation on James-Lange theory." *Psychological Review*, 101(2), 211–221.

Latva, R., Lehtonen, L., Salmelin, R. K., & Tamminen, T. (2004). "Visiting less than every day: a marker for later behavioral problems in Finnish preterm infants." *Archives of Pediatrics and Adolescent Medicine*, 158(12), 1153–1157.

Lau, C. (2016). "Development of infant oral feeding skills: what do we know?" *American Journal of Clinical Nutrition*, 103(Suppl), 616S–621S.

Lau, C., & Hurst, N. (1999). "Oral feeding in infants." *Current Problems in Pediatrics*, 29(4), 105–124.

Lau, C., Hurst, N. M., Smith, E. O., & Schanler, R. J. (2007). "Ethnic/racial diversity, maternal stress, lactation and very low birthweight infants." *Journal of Perinatology*, 27(7), 399–408.

Lau, C., Alagugurusamy, R., Schanler, R. J., Smith, E. O., & Shulman, R. J. (2000). "Characterization of the developmental stages of sucking in preterm infants during bottle feeding." *Acta Paediatrica*, 89(7), 846–852.

Lavelli, M., & Fogel, A. (2005). "Developmental changes in the relationship between infant's attention and emotion during early face-to-face communication: the 2-month transition." *Developmental Psychology*, 41(1), 265–280.

Lawrence, J., Alcock, D., McGrath, P., Kay, J., MacMurray, S. B., & Dulberg, C. (1993). "The development of a tool to assess neonatal pain." *Neonatal Network*, 12(6), 59–66.

Leader, L. R., Baillie, P., Martin, B., & Vermeulen, E. (1982). "The assessment and significance of habituation to a repeated stimulus by the human fetus." *Early Human Development*, 7(3), 211–219.

Lean, R. E., Smyser, C. D., & Rogers, C. E. (2017). "Assessment: the newborn." *Child and Adolescent Psychiatric Clinics of North America*, 26(3), 427–440.

Lee, G. Y., & Kisilevsky, B. S. (2014). "Fetuses respond to father's voice but prefer mother's voice after birth." *Developmental Psychobiology*, 56(1), 1–11.

Lee, J., Kim, H. S., Jung, Y. H., Choi, K. Y., Shin, S. H., Kim, E. K., & Choi, J. H. (2015). "Oropharyngeal colostrum administration in extremely premature infants: an RCT." *Pediatrics*, 135(2), e357–366.

Leentjens, A. F. G., Schieveld, J. N. M., Leonard, M., Lousberg, R., Verhey, F. R. J., & Maegher, D. J. (2008). "A comparison of the phenomenology of pediatric, adult, and geriatric delirium." *Journal of Psychosomatic Research*, 64(2), 219–223.

Lepage, J. F., & Théoret, H. (2007). "The mirror neuron system: grasping others' actions from birth?" *Developmental Science*, 10(5), 513–523.

Levinas, E. (1969). *Totality and Infinity: An Essay on Exteriority*. (A. Lingis, transl.) Pittsburgh, PA: Duquesne University Press. (Original work published 1961).

Levy, D. M. (1928). "Finger sucking and accessory movements in early infancy." *American Journal of Psychiatry*, 84(6), 881–918.

Lewis, C. T., Short, C., & Andrews, E. A. (1879). *Harpers' Latin Dictionary: A New Latin Dictionary Founded on the Translation of Freund's Latin-German Lexicon, Ed. By E. A Andrews, LL. D.* New York, NY: American Book Company.

Ley, P., Bottari, D., Shenoy, B. H., Kekunnaya, R., & Röder, B. (2013). "Partial recovery of visual–spatial remapping of touch after restoring vision in a congenitally blind man." *Neuropsychologia*, 51(6), 1119–1123.

Liu, W. F. (2012). "Comparing sound measurements in the single-family room with open-unit design neonatal intensive care unit: the impact of equipment noise." *Journal of Perinatology*, 32(5), 368–373.

Lyngstad, L. T., Tandberg, B. S., Storm, H., Ekeberg, B. L., & Moen, A. (2014). "Does skin-to-skin contact reduce stress during diaper change in preterm infants?" *Early Human Development*, 90(4), 169–172.

Madlinger-Lewis, L., Reynolds, L., Zarem, C., Crapnell, T., Inder, T., & Pineda, R. (2014). "The effects of alternative positioning on preterm infants in the neonatal intensive care unit: a randomized clinical trial." *Research in Developmental Disabilities*, 35(2), 490–497.

Makói, Z., Szöke, Z., Sasvári, L., Kiss, G., & Popper, P. (1975). "The first cry of the newborn following vaginal delivery or cesarean section." *Acta Paediatrica Academiae Scientiarum Hungaricae*, 16(2), 155–161.

Manganaro, R., Mamì, C., Palmara, A., Paolata, A., & Gemelli, M. (2001). "Incidence of meconium aspiration syndrome in term meconium-stained babies managed at birth with selective tracheal intubation." *Journal of Perinatal Medicine*, 29(6), 465–468.

Marion, J-L. (2002). *In Excess: Studies of Saturated Phenomenon*. (R. Horner, V. Berrand, transl.) New York, NY: Fordham University Press. (Original work published 2001).

Marlier, L., & Schaal, B. (2005). "Human newborns prefer human milk: conspecific milk odor is attractive without postnatal exposure." *Child Development*, 76(1), 155–168.

Marlier, L., Schaal, B., & Soussignan, R. (1998). "Neonatal responsiveness to the odor of amniotic and lacteal fluids: a test of perinatal chemosensory continuity." *Child Development*, 69(3), 611–623.

Marlier, L., Gaugler, C., Astruc, D., & Messer, J. (2007). "La sensibilité olfactive du nouveau-né prématuré" [The olfactory sensitivity of the premature newborn]. *Archives De Pédiatrie*, 14(1), 45–53.

Martin, E., Joeri, P., Loenneker, T., Ekatodramis, D., Vitacco, D., Hennig, J., & Marcar, V. L. (1999). "Visual processing in infants and children studied using functional MRI." *Pediatric Research*, 46(2), 135–140.

Marx, V., & Nagy, E. (2015). "Fetal behavioural responses to maternal voice and touch." *PLoS ONE*, 10(6), e0129118.

Mason, S. J., Harris, G., & Blissett, J. (2005). "Tube feeding in infancy: implications for the development of normal eating and drinking skills." *Dysphagia*, 20(1), 46–61.

Mathai, S., Natrajan, N., & Rajalakshmi, N. R. (2006). "A comparative study of non pharmacological methods to reduce pain in neonates." *Indian Pediatrics*, 43(12), 1070–1075.

Mathew, O. P., Clark, M. L., & Pronske, M. H. (1985). "Apnea, bradycardia, and cyanosis during oral feeding in term neonates." *Journal of Pediatrics*, 106(5), 857.

McCurren, C., & Cronin, S. N. (2003). "Delirium: elders tell their stories and guide nursing practice." *MEDSURG Nursing*, 12(5), 318–423.

McGinnis, K., Murray, E., Cherven, B., McCracken, C., & Travers, C. (2016). "Effect of vibration on pain response to heel lance." *Advances in Neonatal Care*, 16(6), 439–448.

McGowan, J. S., Marsh, R. R., Fowler, S. M., Levy, S. E., & Stallings, V. A. (1991). "Developmental patterns of normal nutritive sucking in infants." *Developmental Medicine and Child Neurology*, 33(10), 891–897.

McPherson, C., & Grunau, R. E. (2014). "Neonatal pain control and neurologic effects of anesthetics and sedatives in preterm infants." *Clinics in Perinatology*, 41(1), 209–227.

Mellor, D. J., Diesch, T. J., Gunn, A. J., & Bennet, L. (2005). "The importance of 'awareness' for understanding fetal pain." *Brain Research Reviews*, 49(3), 455–471.

Melnyk, B. M., Crean, H. F., Feinstein, N. F., & Fairbanks, E. (2008). "Maternal anxiety and depression after a premature infant's discharge from the neonatal intensive care unit: explanatory effects of the creating opportunities for parent empowerment program." *Nursing Research*, 57(6), 383–394.

Meltzoff, A. N. (1999). "Origins of theory of mind, cognition and communication." *Journal of Communication Disorders*, 32(4), 251–269.

Meltzoff, A. N., & Moore, M. K. (1977). "Imitation of facial and manual gestures by human neonates." *Science*, 198(4312), 75–78.

Meltzoff, A. N., & Moore, M. K. (1983). "Newborn infants imitate adult facial gestures." *Child Development*, 54(3), 702–709.

Meltzoff, A. N., & Moore, M. K. (1994). "Imitation, memory, and the representation of persons." *Infant Behavior and Development*, 17(1), 83–99.

Meltzoff, A. N., & Moore, M. K. (1997). "Explaining facial imitation: a theoretical model." *Early Development and Parenting*, 6(3–4), 179–192.

Mennella, J. A. (2007). "The chemical senses and the development of flavor preferences in humans." In: T. W. Hale & P. E. Hartmann (eds.), *Hale & Hartmann's Textbook of Human Lactation*. Amarillo, TX: Hale Publishing. pp. 403–414.

Mercuri, E., Baranello, G., Romeo, D. M. M., Cesarini, L., & Ricci, D. (2007). "The development of vision." *Early Human Development*, 83(12), 795–800.

Merleau-Ponty, M. (1962). *Phenomenology of Perception*. (C. Smith, transl.) London: Routledge & Kegan Paul Ltd. (Original work published 1945).

Merleau-Ponty, M. (1963). *The Structure of Behavior*. (A. L. Fisher, transl.) Boston, MA: Beacon Press. (Original work published 1942).

Merleau-Ponty, M. (1964a). "Phenomenology and the sciences of man." (J. Wild, transl.) In: J. M. Edie (ed.), *The Primacy of Perception and Other Essays on Phenomenological Psychology, the Philosophy of Art, History and Politics*. Evanston, IL: Northwestern University Press. pp. 43–95. (Original work published 1961).

Merleau-Ponty, M. (1964b). *Signs*. (R. C. McCleary, transl.) Evanston, IL: Northwestern University Press. (Original work published 1960).

Merleau-Ponty, M. (1964c). *Sense and Non-Sense.* (H. L. Dreyfus, P. A. Dreyfus, transl.) Evanston, IL: Northwestern University Press. (Original work published 1948).

Merleau-Ponty, M. (1968). *The Visible and the Invisible.* (A. Lingis, transl.) Evanston, IL: Northwestern University Press. (Original work published 1964).

Merleau-Ponty, M. (2007). "The child's relations with others." (J. Wild, transl.) In: T. Toadvine & L. Lawlor (eds.), *The Merleau-Ponty Reader.* Evanston, IL: Northwestern University Press. pp. 143–183. (Original work published 1951).

Merleau-Ponty, M. (2010). *Child Psychology and Pedagogy: The Sorbonne Lectures 1949–1952.* (T. Welsh, transl.) Evanston, IL: Northwestern University Press. (Original work published 2001).

MessingerD. S., & Fogel, A. (2007). "The interactive development of social smiling." In: R. V. Kail (ed.), *Advances in Child Development and Behavior.* Cambridge, MA: Elsevier Inc. pp. 327–366.

Messinger, D. S., Fogel, A., & Dickson, K. L. (1999). "What's in a smile?" *Developmental Psychology,* 35(3), 701–708.

Messinger, D. S., Fogel, A., & Dickson, K. L. (2001). "All smiles are positive, but some smiles are more positive." *Developmental Psychology,* 37(5), 642–653.

Messinger, D. S., Dondi, M., Nelson-Goens, G. C., Beghi, A., Fogel, A., & Simion, F. (2002). "How sleeping neonates smile." *Developmental Science,* 5(1), 48–54.

Michelsson, K., & Michelsson, O. (1999). "Phonation in the newborn, infant cry." *International Journal of Pediatric Otorhinolaryngology,* 49(Supp 1), S297–S301.

Michelsson, K., Eklund, K., Leppänen, P., & Lyytinen, H. (2002). "Cry characteristics of 172 healthy 1- to 7-day-old infants." *Folia Phoniatrica et Logopaedica,* 54(4), 190–200.

Miles, M. S., Funk, S. G., & Carlson, J. (1993). "Parental stressor scale: neonatal intensive care unit." *Nursing Research,* 42(3), 148–152.

Miller, J. L., Sonies, B. C., & Macedonia, C. (2003). "Emergence of oropharyngeal, laryngeal and swallowing activity in the developing fetal upper aerodigestive tract: an ultrasound evaluation." *Early Human Development,* 71(1), 61–87.

Miller, M. J., & DiFiore, J. M. (1995). "A comparison of swallowing during apnea and periodic breathing in premature infants." *Pediatric Research,* 37(6), 796–799.

Mirmiran, M., & Ariagno, R. L. (2000). "Influence of light in the NICU on the development of circadian rhythms in preterm infants." *Seminars in Perinatology,* 24(4), 247–257.

Monteagudo, B., & León-Muiños, E. (2010). "Neonatal sucking blisters." *Indian Pediatrics,* 47(9), 794.

Moore, E. R., Bergman, N., Anderson, G. C., & Medley, N. (2016). "Early skin-to-skin contact for mothers and their healthy newborn infants." *Cochrane Database of Systematic Reviews,* 11, CD003519.

Moore, L. M., Persaud, T. V. N., & Torchia, M. G. (2015). *The Developing Human: Clinical Oriented Embryology.* Philadelphia, PA: Saunders.

Morton, J., & Johnson, M. H. (1991). "CONSPEC and CONLERN: a two-process theory of infant face recognition." *Psychological Review,* 98(2), 164–181.

Myowa-Yamakoshi, M., & Takeshita, H. (2006). "Do human fetuses anticipate self-oriented actions? A study by four-dimensional (4D) ultrasonography." *Infancy,* 10(3), 289–301.

Nagy, E. (2008). "Innate intersubjectivity: newborns' sensitivity to communication disturbance." *Developmental Psychology,* 44(6), 1779–1784.

Nagy, E., Kompagne, H., Orvos, H., & Pal, A. (2007). "Gender related differences in neonatal imitation." *Infant and Child Development,* 16(3), 267–276.

Nagy, E., Kompagne, H., Orvos, H., Pal, A., Molnar, P., Janszky, I., & Bardos, G. (2005). "Index finger movement imitation by human neonates: motivation, learning, and left-hand preference." *Pediatric Research*, 58(4), 749–753.

Nelson, J. K. (2005). *Seeing Through Tears: Crying and Attachment*. New York, NY: Brunner-Routledge.

Newman, J. D. (2007). "Neural circuits underling crying and cry responding in mammals." *Behavioural Brain Research*, 182(2), 155–165.

Nilsson, L. (1973). *Behold Man: A Photographic Journey of Discovery Inside the Body*. Boston, MA: Little, Brown.

O'Donnell, C. P., Kamlin, C. O., Davis, P. G., & Morley, C. J. (2010). "Crying and breathing by extremely preterm infants immediately after birth." *Journal of Pediatrics*, 156 (5), 846–847.

O'Malley, G., Leonard, M., Maegher, D., & O'Keeffe, S. T. (2008). "The delirium experience: a review." *Journal of Psychosomatic Research*, 65(3), 223–228.

Ockleford, E. M., Vince, M. A., Layton, C., & Reader, M. R. (1988). "Responses of neonates to parents' and others' voices." *Early Human Development*, 18(1), 27–36.

Oster, H. (1978). "Facial expression and affect development." In: M. Lewis & L. A. Rosenblum (eds.), *The Development of Affect*. New York, NY: Plenum Press. pp. 43–75.

Ostwald, P. (1972). "The sounds of infancy." *Developmental Medicine & Child Neurology*, 14 (3), 350–361.

Parvizi, J., Coburn, K. L., Shillcutt, S. D., Coffey, C. E., Lauterbach, E. C., & Mendez, M. F. (2009). "Neuroanatomy of pathological laughing and crying: a report of the American Neuropsychiatric Association Committee on Research." *Journal of Neuropsychiatry and Clinical Neurosciences*, 21(1), 75–87.

Patrick, J., Campbell, K., Carmichael, L., Natale, R., & Richardson, B. (1982). "Patterns of gross foetal body movements over 24-hour observation intervals during the last 10 weeks of pregnancy." *Obstetrics & Gynecology*, 142(4), 363–371.

Petrikovsky, B. M., Kaplan, G., & Holsten, N. (2003). "Eyelid movements in normal human fetuses." *Journal of Clinical Ultrasound*, 31(6), 299–301.

Piaget, J. (1950). *The Psychology of Intelligence*. San Diego, CA: Harcourt Brace Jovanovich.

Pillai, M., & James, D. (1990). "Are the behavioural states of the newborn comparable to those of the foetus?" *Early Human Development*, 22(1), 39–49.

Pineda, R., Guth, R., Herring, A., Reynolds, L., Oberle, S., & Smith, J. (2017). "Enhancing sensory experiences for very preterm infants in the NICU: an integrative review." *Journal of Perinatology*, 37(4), 323–332.

Pineda, R. G., Neil, J., Dierker, D., Smyser, C. D., Wallendorf, M., Kidokoro, H., Reynolds, L. C., Walker, S., Rogers, C., Mathur, A. M., Van Essen, D. C., & Inder, T. (2014). "Alterations in brain structure and neurodevelopmental outcome in preterm infants hospitalized in different neonatal intensive care environments." *Journal of Pediatrics*, 164(1), 52–60.e2.

Pinelli, J., & Symington, A. (2005). "Non-nutritive sucking for promoting physiologic stability and nutrition in preterm infants." *Cochrane Database of Systematic Reviews*, 4, CD001071

Pinyerd, B. J. (1994). "Infant cries: physiology and assessment." *Neonatal Network*, 13(4), 15–20.

Piontelli, A. (2010) *Development of Normal Fetal Movements: The First 25 Weeks of Gestation*. Milan: Springer-Verlag.

Platt, M. W. (2011). "Fetal awareness and fetal pain: the emperor's new clothes." *Archives of Disease in Childhood. Fetal and Neonatal Edition*, 96(4), F236–237.

Plessner, H. (1970). *Laughing and Crying: A Study of the Limits of Human Behaviour*. Evanston, IL: Northwestern University Press.

Potter, E. (1946). "Bilateral renal agenesis." *Journal of Pediatrics*, 29, 68–76.

Querleu, D., Renard, X., Boutteville, C., & Crepin, G. (1989). "Hearing by the human fetus?" *Seminars in Perinatology*, 13(5), 409–420.

Raes, J., Michelsson, K., Dehaen, F., & Despontin, M. (1982). "Cry analysis in infants with infectious and congenital disorders of the larynx." *International Journal of Pediatric Otorhinolaryngology*, 4(2), 157–169.

Ramenghi, L. A., Ricci, D., Mercuri, E., Groppo, M., De Carli, A., Ometto, A., Fumagalli, M., Bassi, L., Pisoni, S., Cioni, G., & Mosca, F. (2010). "Visual performance and brain structures in the developing brain of pre-term infants." *Early Human Development*, 86 (Suppl 1), S73–S75.

Ranger, M., Johnston, C. C., & Anand, K. J. S. (2007). "Current controversies regarding pain assessment in neonates." *Seminars in Perinatology*, 31(5), 283–288.

Ranger, M., Synnes, A. R., Vinall, J., & Grunau, R. E. (2014). "Internalizing behaviours in school-age children born very preterm are predicted by neonatal pain and morphine exposure." *European Journal of Pain*, 18(6), 844–852.

Ranger, M., Chau, C. M., Garg, A., Woodward, T. S., Beg, M. F., Bjornson, B., Poskitt, K., Fitzpatrick, K., Synnes, A. R., Miller, S. P., & Grunau, R. E. (2013). "Neonatal pain-related stress predicts cortical thickness at age 7 years in children born very pre-term." *PLoS ONE*, 8(10), e76702.

Rattaz, C., Goubet, N., & Bullinger, A. (2005). "The calming effect of a familiar odor on full-term newborns." *Journal of Developmental and Behavioral Pediatrics*, 26(2), 86–92.

Reissland, N. (1988). "Neonatal imitation in the first hour of life: observation in rural Nepal." *Developmental Psychology*, 24(4), 464–469.

Reissland, N., Francis, B., Aydin, E., Mason, J., & Schaal, B. (2014). "The development of anticipation in the fetus: a longitudinal account of human fetal mouth movements in reaction to and anticipation of touch." *Developmental Psychobiology*, 56(5), 955–963.

Reynolds, L. C., Duncan, M. M., Smith, G. C., Mathur, A., Neil, J., Inder, T., & Pineda, R. G. (2013). "Parental presence and holding in the neonatal intensive care unit and associations with early neurobehavior." *Journal of Perinatology*, 33(8), 636–641.

Ricci, D., Romeo, D. M., Gallini, F., Groppo, M., Cesarini, L., Pisoni, S., Serrao, F., Papacci, P., Contaldo, I., Perrino, F., Brogna, C., Bianco, F., Baranello, G., Sacco, A., Quintiliani, M., Ornetto, A., Cilauro, S., Mosca, F., Romagnoli, C., Romeo, M. G., Cowan, F., Cioni, G., Ramenghi, L., & Mercuri, E. (2011). "Early visual assessment in preterm infants with and without brain lesions: correlation with visual and neurodevelopmental outcome at 12 months." *Early Human Development*, 87(3), 177–182.

Ricoeur, P. (1966). *Freedom and Nature: The Voluntary and the Involuntary*. (E. V. Kohák, Trans.). Evanston, IL: Northwestern University Press. (Original work published 1950).

Righard, L., & Blade, M. O. (1994) "Effect of delivery routines on success of first breast-feed." *Lancet*, 336(8723), 1105–1107.

Robb, M. P., & Cacace, A. T. (1995). "Estimation of formant frequencies in infant cry." *International Journal of Pediatric Otorhinolaryngology*, 32(1), 57–67.

Roberts, A. B., Little, D., Cooper, D., & Campbell, S. (1979). "Normal patterns of fetal activity in the third trimester." *British Journal of Obstetrics and Gynaecology*, 86(1), 4–9.

Rochat, P. (1993). "Hand-mouth coordination in the newborn: morphology, determinants, and early development of a basic act." In: G. J. P. Savelsbergh (ed.), *The Development of Coordination in Infancy*. Amsterdam: North-Holland/Elsevier. pp. 265–288.

Rochat, P. (2001). *The Infant's World*. Cambridge, MA: Harvard University Press.

Rochat, P. (2003). "Five levels of self-awareness as they unfold early in life." *Consciousness and Cognition*, 12(4), 717–731.

Rochat, P., & Hespos, S. J. (1997). "Differential rooting response by neonates: evidence for an early sense of self." *Early Development and Parenting*, 6(3–4), 105–112.

Rochat, P., Blass, M., & Hoffmeyer, L. B. (1988). "Oropharyngeal control of hand-mouth coordination in newborn infants." *Developmental Psychology*, 24(4), 459–463.

Roes, F. L. (1989). "On the origin of crying and tears." *Human Ethology Newsletter*, 5(10), 5–6.

Romano, C. (2015). *At the Heart of Reason*. (M. B. Smith, C. Romano, transl.) Evanston, IL: Northwestern University Press. (Original work published 2010).

Rosen, C. L., Glaze, D. G., & Frost, J. D. Jr. (1984). "Hypoxemia associated with feeding in the preterm infant and full-term neonate." *American Journal of Diseases of Children*, 138 (7), 623–628.

Rovee, C. K., & Levin, G. R. (1966). "Oral 'pacification' and arousal in the human newborn." *Journal of Experimental Child Psychology*, 3(1), 1–17.

Rudolph, A. M., Iwamoto, H. S., & Teitel, D. F. (1988). "Circulatory changes at birth." *Journal of Perinatal Medicine*, 16(suppl 1), 9–21.

Russell, P. M. (1957). "Vagitus uterinus; crying in utero." *Lancet*, 272(6960), 137–138.

Sadler, T. W. (2015). *Langman's Medical Embryology*. Philadelphia, PA: Wolters Kluwer Health.

Salk, L. (1973). "The role of the heartbeat in the relation between mother and infant." *Scientific American*, 228(5), 24–29.

Sandman, C. A., Davis, E. P., Buss, C., & Glynn, L. M. (2012). "Exposure to prenatal psychobiological stress exerts programming influences on the mother and her fetus." *Neuroendocrinology*, 95(1), 7–21.

Sann, C., & Streri, A. (2007). "Perception of object shape and texture in human newborns: evidence from cross-modal transfer tasks." *Developmental Science*, 10(3), 399–410.

Santos, J., Pearce, S. E., & Stroustrup, A. (2015). "Impact of hospital-based environmental exposures on neurodevelopmental outcomes of preterm infants." *Current Opinion in Pediatrics*, 27(2), 254–260.

Sartre, J.-P. (1956). *Being and Nothingness: A Phenomenological Essay on Ontology*. (H. E. Barnes, transl.) New York, NY: Philosophical Library. (Original work published 1943).

Sartre, J.-P. (1991). *The Transcendence of the Ego: An Existentialist Theory of Consciousness*. (F. Williams, R. Kirkpatrick, transl.) New York, NY: Hill & Wang. (Original work published 1937).

Scanlon J. (1985). "Barbarism in the nursery." *Perinatal Press*, 9(7), 103–104.

Schaal, B., Hummel, T., & Soussignan, R. (2004). "Olfaction in the fetal and premature infant: functional status and clinical implications." *Clinical Perinatology*, 31(2), 261–285.

Schaal, B., Marlier, L., & Soussignan, R. (1998). "Olfactory function in the human fetus: evidence from selective neonatal responsiveness to the odor of amniotic fluid." *Behavioral Neuroscience*, 112(6), 1438–1449.

Schanler, R. J., Shulman, R. J., Lau, C., Smith, E. O., & Heitkemper, M. M. (1999). "Feeding strategies for premature infants: randomized trial of gastrointestinal priming and tube-feeding method." *Pediatrics*, 103(2), 434–439.

Scheler, M. (1954). *The Nature of Sympathy*. (P. Heath, transl.) London: Routledge & Kegan Paul. (Original work published 1913).

Schloim, N., Vereijken, C. M., Blundell, P., & Hetherington, M. M. (2016). "Looking for cues – infant communication of hunger and satiation during milk feeding." *Appetite*, 108, 74–82.

Schoenfeld, M. A., Neuer, G., Tempelmann, C., Schüssler, K., Noesselt, T., Hopf, J. M., & Heinze, H. J. (2004). "Functional magnetic resonance tomography correlates of taste perception in the human primary taste cortex." *Neuroscience*, 127(2), 347–353.

Schofield, I. (1997). "A small exploratory study of the reaction of older people to an episode of delirium." *Journal of Advanced Nursing*, 25(5), 942–952.

Schwab, M., Bludau, T., Abrams, R. M., Antonelli, P. J., Gerhard, K. J., & Bauer, R. (1997). "Thermal stimulation of the fetal skin induces ECoG arousal in fetal sheep." *Pflugers Archiv: European Journal of Physiology*, 433(6), 594.

Seidman, G., Unnikrishnan, S., & Kenny, E. (2015). "Barriers and enables of kangaroo mother care practice: a systematic review." *PLoS One*, 10(5), e0125643.

Shahheidari, M., & Homer, C. (2012). "Impact of the design of neonatal intensive care units on neonates, staff, and families: a systemic literature review." *The Journal of Perinatal and Neonatal Nursing*, 26(3), 260–266.

Shu, S. H., Lee, Y. L., Hayter, M., & Wang, R. H. (2014). "Efficacy of swaddling and heel warming on pain response to heel stick in neonates: a randomized control trial." *Journal of Clinical Nursing*, 23(21–22), 3107–3114.

Simms, E. (2008). *The Child in the World: Embodiment, Time, and Language in Early Childhood*. Detroit, MI: Wayne State University Press.

Simons, S. H., van Dijk, M., Anand, K. S., Roofthooft, D., van Lingen, R. A., & Tibboel, D. (2003). "Do we still hurt newborn babies? A prospective study of procedural pain and analgesia in neonates." *Archives of Pediatrics & Adolescent Medicine*, 157(11), 1058–1064.

Simpson, E. A., Murray, L., Paukner, A., & Ferrari, P. F. (2014). "The mirror neuron system as revealed through neonatal imitation: presence from birth, predictive power and evidence of plasticity." *Philosophical Transactions of the Royal Society B: Biological Sciences*, 369, 20130289.

Slater, A., Brown, E., & Badenoch, M. (1997). "Intermodal perception at birth: newborn infants' memory for arbitrary auditory–visual pairings." *Early Development and Parenting*, 6(3–4), 99–104.

Slater, R., Fabrizi, L., Worley, A., Meek, J., Boyd, S., & Fitzgerald, M. (2010a). "Premature infants display increased noxious evoked neuronal activity in the brain compared to healthy age-matched term-born infants." *NeuroImage*, 52(2), 583–589.

Slater, R., Cantarella, A., Gallella, S., Worley, A., Boyd, S., Meek, J., & Fitzgerald, M. (2006). "Cortical pain responses in human infants." *Journal of Neuroscience*, 26(14), 3662–3666.

Slater, R., Worley, A., Fabrizi, L., Roberts, S., Meek, J., Boyd, S., & Fitzgerald, M. (2010b). "Evoked potentials generated by noxious stimulation in the human infant brain." *European Journal of Pain*, 14(3), 321–326.

Smith, C. V., Satt, B., Phelan, J. P., & Paul, R. H. (1990). "Intrauterine sound levels: intrapartum assessment with an intrauterine microphone." *American Journal of Perinatology*, 7(4), 312–315.

Smith, G. C., Gutovich, J., Smyser, C., Pineda, R., Newnham, C., Tjoeng, T. H., Vavasseur, C., Wallendorf, M., Neil, J., & Inder, T. (2011). "Neonatal intensive care unit stress is associated with brain development in preterm infants." *Annals of Neurology*, 70(4), 541–549.

Smith, J. R. (2012). "Comforting touch in the very preterm hospitalized infant: an integrative review." *Advances in Neonatal Care*, 12(6), 349–365.

Soussignan, R., Schaal, B., Marlier, L., & Jiang, T. (1997). "Facial and autonomic responses to biological and artificial olfactory stimuli in human neonates: re-examining early hedonic discrimination of odors." *Physiology and Behavior*, 62(4), 745–758.

Spiecker, B. (1984). "The pedagogical relationship." *Oxford Review of Education*, 10(2), 203–209.

Standley, J. M. (2001). "Music therapy for the neonate." *Newborn and Infant Nursing Reviews*, 1(4), 211–216.

Stein, E. (1989). *On the Problem of Empathy*. (W. Stein, transl.) Washington, DC: ICS Publications. (Original work published 1917).

Steinhorn, R., McPherson, C., Anderson, P. J., Neil, J., Doyle, L. W., & Inder, T. (2015). "Neonatal morphine exposure in very preterm infants—cerebral development and outcomes." *Journal of Pediatrics*, 166(5), 1200–1207.

Stenwall, E., Jonhagen, M. E., Sandberg, J., & Fagerberg, I. (2008). "The older patient's experience of encountering professional carers and close relatives during an acute confusional state: an interview study." *International Journal of Nursing Studies*, 45(11), 1577–1585.

Stern, D. N. (1985). *The Interpersonal World of the Infant: A View from Psychoanalysis and Developmental Psychology*. New York, NY: Basic Books.

Stevens, B., Johnston, C., Petryshen, P., & Taddio, A. (1996). "Premature Infant Pain Profile: development and initial validation." *Clinical Journal of Pain*, 12(1), 13–22.

Stevens, B., Yamada, J., Ohlsson, A.Haliburton, S., & Shorkey, A. (2016). "Sucrose for analgesia in newborn infants undergoing painful procedures." *Cochrane Database of Systematic Reviews*, 7, CD001069.

Stevens, D., Thompson, P., Helseth, C., & Pottala, J. (2015). "Mounting evidence favoring single-family room neonatal intensive care." *Journal of Neonatal Perinatal Medicine*, 8 (3), 177–178.

Stjerna, S., Sairanen, V., Gröhn, R., Andersson, S., Metsäranta, M., Lano, A., & Vanhatalo, S. (2015). "Visual fixation in human newborns correlates with extensive white matter networks and predicts long-term neurocognitive development." *The Journal of Neuroscience*, 35(12), 4824–4829.

Stoerig, P., & Cowey, A. (1997). "Blindsight in man and monkey." *Brain*, 120(Pt 3), 535–559.

Streri, A., de Hevia, M. D., Izard, V., & Coubart, A. (2013). "What do we know about neonatal cognition." *Behavioral Sciences*, 3(1), 154–169.

Struyker Boudier, C. E. M. (1986). "Merleau-Ponty and Buytendijk: report of a relationship." (R. Rojcewicz, transl.) In: S. Strasser (ed.), *Clefts in the World and Other Essays on Levinas, Merleau-Ponty, and Buytendijk*. Pittsburgh, PA: The Simon Silverman Phenomenology Center Duquesne University. pp. 1–27.

Surenthiran, S. S., Wilbraham, K., May, J., Chant, T., Emmerson, A. J., & Newton, V. E. (2013). "Noise levels within the ear and post-nasal space in neonates in intensive care." *Archives of Disease in Childhood. Fetal and Neonatal Edition*, 88(4), F315–F318.

Swain, J. E., Lorberbaum, J. P., Kose, S., & Strathearn, L. (2007). "Brain basis of early parent–infant interactions: psychology, physiology, and in vivo functional neuroimaging studies." *Journal of Child Psychology and Psychiatry*, 48(3–4), 262–287.

Tawfik, H. A., Abdulhafez, M. H., Fouad, Y. A., & Dutton, J. J. (2016). "Embryologic and fetal development of the human eyelid." *Ophthalmic Plastic and Reconstructive Surgery*, 32(6), 407–414.

Te Pas, A. B., Wong, C., Kamlin, C. O., Dawson, J. A., Morley, C. J., & Davis, P. G. (2009). "Breathing patterns in preterm and term infants immediately after birth." *Pediatric Research*, 65(3), 352–356.

Teitel, D. F., Iwamoto, H. S., & Rudolph, A. M. (1990). "Changes in the pulmonary circulation during birth-related events." *Pediatric Research*, 27(4 Pt 1), 372–378.

Thakkar, P., Arora, K., Goyal, K., Das, R. R., Javadekar, B., Aiyer, S., & Panigrahi, S. K. (2016). "To evaluate and compare the efficacy of combined sucrose and non-nutritive sucking for analgesia in newborns undergoing minor painful procedure: a randomized controlled trial." *Journal of Perinatology*, 36(1), 67–70.

Traube, C., Silver, G., Kearney, J., Patel, A., Atkinson, T. M., Yoon, M. J., Halpert, S., Augenstein, J., Sickles, L. E., Li, C., & Greenwald, B. (2014). "Cornell assessment of pediatric delirium: a valid, rapid, observational tool for screening delirium in the PICU." *Critical Care Medicine*, 42(3), 656–663.

Trevarthen, C., & Aitken, C. (2003). "Regulation of brain development and age-related changes in infants' motives: the developmental function of regressive periods." In: M. Heimann (ed.), *Regression Periods in Human Infancy*. Mahwah, NJ: Erlbaum. pp. 107–184.

Turkel, S. B., Trzepacz, P. T., & Tavare, C. J. (2006). "Comparing symptoms of delirium in adults and children." *Psychosomatics*, 47(4), 320–324.

Uga, E., Candriella, M., Perino, A., Alloni, V., Angilella, G., Trada, M., Ziliotto, A. M., Rossi, M. B., Tozzini, D., Tripaldi, C., Vaglio, M., Grossi, L., Allen, M., & Provera, S. (2008). "Heel lance in newborn during breastfeeding: an evaluation of analgesic effect of this procedure." *Italian Journal of Pediatrics*, 34(1), 3.

Unruh, A. M. (1992). "Voices from the past: ancient views of pain in childhood." *Clinical Journal of Pain*, 8(3), 247–254.

Valman, H. B., & Pearson, J. F. (1980). "What the fetus feels." *British Medical Journal, 280* (6209), 233–234.

Van den Berg, J. H. (1966). *The Psychology of the Sickbed*. New York, NY: Duquesne University Press. (Original work published 1959).

Van Manen, M. (1990). *Researching Lived Experience: Human Science for an Action Sensitive Pedagogy*. Albany, NY: SUNY Press; London, ON: Althouse Press.

Van Manen, M. (2001). "Professional practice and 'doing phenomenology.'" In: S. Kay Toombs (ed.), *Handbook of Phenomenology and Medicine (Philosophy and Medicine Series)*. Dordrecht: Kluwer Press. pp. 457–474.

Van Manen, M. (2014). *Phenomenology of Practice: Meaning-Giving Methods in Phenomenological Research and Writing*. Walnut Creek, CA: Left Coast Press.

Van Manen, M. A. (2012). "Technics of touch in the neonatal intensive care." *Medical Humanities*, 38(2), 91–96.

Van Vonderen, J. J., Roest, A. A., Walther, F. J., Blom, N. A., van Lith, J. M., Hooper, S. B., & te Pas, A. B. (2015). "The influence of crying on the ductus arteriosus shunt and left ventricular output at birth." *Neonatology*, 107(2), 108–112.

Van Vonderen, J. J., te Pas, A. B., Kolster-Bijdevaate, C., van Lith, J. M., Blom, N. A., Hooper, S. B., & Roest, A. A. (2014). "Non-invasive measurements of ductus arteriosus flow directly after birth." *Archives of Disease in Childhood. Fetal and Neonatal Edition*, 99 (5), F408–F412.

Varendi, H., & Porter, R. H. (2001). "Breast odour as the only maternal stimulus elicits crawling towards the odour source." *Acta Paediatrica*, 90(4), 372–375.

Varendi, H., Porter, R. H., & WinbergJ. (1994). "Does the newborn baby find the nipple by smell?" *Lancet*, 344(8928), 989–990.

Varendi, H., Porter, R. H., & Winberg, J. (1996). "Attractiveness of amniotic fluid odor: evidence of prenatal olfactory learning?" *Acta Paediatrica*, 85(10), 1223–1227.

Varendi, H., Christensson, K., Porter, R. H., & Winberg, J. (1998). "Soothing effect of amniotic fluid smell in newborn infants." *Early Human Development*, 51(1), 47–55.

Velmans, M., & Schneider, S. (eds.). (2007). *The Blackwell Companion to Consciousness*. Malden, MA: Wiley-Blackwell.

Vergara, E. R., & Bigsby, R. (2004). *Developmental and Therapeutic Interventions in the NICU*. Baltimore, MD: Paul H. Brookes Publishing Company.

Verriotis, M., Fabrizi, L., Lee, A., Ledwidge, S., Meek, J., & Fitzgerald, M. (2015). "Cortical activity evoked by inoculation needle prick in infants up to one-year old." *PAIN*, 156(2), 222–230.

Vinall, J., Miller, S. P., Bjornson, B. H., Fitzpatrick, K. P., Poskitt, K. J., Brant, R., Synnes, A. R., Cepeda, I. L., & Grunau, R. E. (2014). "Invasive procedures in preterm children: brain and cognitive development at school age." *Pediatrics*, 133(3), 412–421.

Vingerhoets, A. D. (2013). *Why Only Humans Weep: Unravelling the Mysteries of Tears*. Oxford: Oxford University Press.

Vingerhoets, A. J. J. M., Cornelius, R. R., van Heck, G. L., & Becht, M. C. (2000). "Adult crying: a model and review of the literature." *Review of General Psychology*, 4(4), 354–377.

Voegtline, K. M., Costigan, K. A., Pater, H. A., & DiPietro, J. A. (2013). "Near-term fetal response to maternal spoken voice." *Infant Behavior and Development*, 36(4), 526–533.

Vuilleumier, P., Armony, J. L., Driver, J., & Dolan, R. J. (2003). "Distinct spatial frequency sensitivities for processing faces and emotional expressions." *Nature Neuroscience*, 6(6), 624–631.

Waldenfels, B. (2007). *The Question of the Other*. Hong Kong: The Chinese University Press.

Walker, H. K. (1990). "The suck, snout, palmomental, and grasp reflexes." In: H. K. Walker, W. D. Hall & J. W. Hurst (eds.), *Clinical Methods: The History, Physical, and Laboratory Examinations*. Boston, MA: Butterworths. pp. 363–364.

Walton, G. E., Bower, N. J., & Bower, T. G. (1992). "Recognition of familiar faces by newborns." *Infant Behavior and Development*, 15(2), 265–269.

Wasz-Hökert, O., Lind, J., Partanem, T., Vallane, E., & Vuorenkoski, V. (1968). "The infant cry: a spectrographic and auditory analysis." *Clinics in Developmental Medicine*, 29, 1–42.

Waterland, R. A., Berkowitz, R. I., Stunkard, A. J., & Stallings, V. A. (1998). "Calibrated orifice nipples for measurement of infant nutritive sucking." *Journal of Pediatrics*, 132(3 Pt 1), 523–526.

Waters, S. F., West, T. V., & Mendes, W. B. (2014). "Stress contagion: physiological covariation between mothers and infants." *Psychological Science*, 25(4), 934–942.

Weiner, G. M. (ed.). (2016). *Textbook of Neonatal Resuscitation, 7th Edition*. Elk Grove Village, IL: American Academy of Pediatrics.

Weiskrantz, L. (1996). "Blindsight revisited." *Current Opinion in Neurobiology*, 6, 215–220.

Wider, K. (1999). "The self and others: imitation in infants and Sartre's analysis of the look." *Continental Philosophy Review*, 32(2), 195–210.

Widström, A.-M., Ransjö-Arvidson, A.-B., Christensson, K., Matthiesen, A.-S., Winberg, J., & Uvnäs-Moberg, K. (1987). "Gastric suction in the newborn infants: effects on circulation and developing feeding behaviours." *Acta Paediatrica Scandinavica*, 76(4), 566–572.

Wilkinson, A. R., & Jiang, Z. D. (2006). "Brainstem auditory evoked response in neonatal neurology." *Seminars in Fetal Neonatal Medicine*, 11(6), 444–451.

Wolff, P. H. (1959). "Observations on newborn infants." *Psychosomatic Medicine*, 21(2), 110–118.

Wolff, P. H. (1968). "The serial organization of sucking in the young infant." *Pediatrics*, 42 (6), 943–956.

Woolridge, M. W. (1986). "The 'anatomy' of infant sucking." *Midwifery*, 2(4), 164–171.

World Health Organization. (2018). Preterm birth. Fact sheet. Updated February 2018. Retrieved from www.who.int/en/news-room/fact-sheets/detail/preterm-birth.

Yan, F., Dai, S. Y., Akther, N., Kuno, A., Yanagihara, T., & Hata, T. (2006). "Four-dimensional sonographic assessment of fetal facial expression early in the third trimester." *International Journal of Gynecology and Obstetrics*, 94(2), 108–113.

Yaster, M. (1987). "Analgesia and anesthesia in neonates." *Journal of Pediatrics*, 111(3), 394–395.

Yong Ping, E., Laplante, D. P., Elgbeili, G., Hillerer, K. M., Brunet, A., O'Hara, M. W., & King, S. (2015). "Prenatal maternal stress predicts stress reactivity at 2 ½ years of age: the Iowa Flood Study." *Psychoneuroendocrinology*, 56, 62–78.

Zahavi, D. (2001). "Beyond empathy: phenomenological approaches to intersubjectivity." *Journal of Consciousness Studies*, 8(5–7), 151–167.

Zahavi, D. (2005). *Subjectivity and Selfhood: Investigating the First-Person Perspective*. Cambridge, MA: MIT Press.

Zahavi, D. (2014). *Self and Other: Exploring Subjectivity, Empathy, and Shame*. Oxford: Oxford University Press.

Zanardo, V., & Straface, G. (2015). "The higher temperature in the areola supports the natural progression of the birth to breastfeeding continuum." *PLoS ONE*, 10(3), e0118774.

Zimmer, E. Z., Chao, C. R., Guy, G. P., Marks, F., & Fifer, W. P. (1993). "Vibroacoustic stimulation evokes human fetal micturition." *Obstetrics and Gynecology*, 81(2), 178–180.

Zwicker, J. G., Miller, S. P., Grunau, R. E., Chau, V., Brant, R., Studholme, C., Lui, M., Synnes, A., Poskitt, K. J., Stiver, M. L., & Tam, E. W. (2016). "Smaller cerebellar growth and poorer neurodevelopmental outcomes in very preterm infants exposed to neonatal morphine." *Journal of Pediatrics*, 172, 81–87.e2.

INDEX